Florence

Florence Nightingale

Catherine Swift

Marshall Pickering
An Imprint of HarperCollins*Publishers*

Marshall Pickering is an Imprint of
HarperCollins*Religious*
Part of HarperCollins*Publishers*
77–85 Fulham Palace Road, London W6 8JB

First published in Great Britain
in 1993 by Marshall Pickering
1 3 5 7 9 10 8 6 4 2

A catalogue record for this book is
available from the British Library

ISBN 0 551 02562–X

Printed and bound in Great Britain by
HarperCollinsManufacturing Glasgow

CONTENTS

1.

NINETEENTH-CENTURY HIGH SOCIETY

The Victorian age is always criticized for the restrictive behaviour patterns it imposed on people – and especially on females. But long before 1837, when Queen Victoria ascended the throne, many of the attitudes now attributed to her reign were in practice.

Women who weren't either married or betrothed by the time they reached their mid-twenties invariably remained unmarried for life. Usually the most unattractive of females, they were labelled "old maids" and fell into the roles of unpaid servants to their parents and as "maiden aunts" to their siblings' children.

So everybody was puzzled when Frances Smith, known affectionately as Fanny – a renowned beauty who was wooed by many suitors – reached the age of thirty before she married.

Even more surprising was that her husband, William Edward Nightingale, known by his initials as WEN, was only twenty-three years old.

It was virtually unknown – even something of a stigma – for the bride to be as much as a few weeks older than the groom, let alone seven years. But then, WEN and Fanny seemed ill-matched individuals in lots of ways.

Both came from wealthy, high-ranking families and were intelligent, popular and physically attractive.

Fanny, however, was a rather shallow character, totally absorbed in frivolous and selfish pursuits, while WEN was shy, quiet and bookish. He loved a peaceful existence and wasn't particularly ambitious. And he didn't need to be. From an uncle, he'd inherited an annual allowance of £8,000, which in those days was a fortune, so he was an extremely wealthy young man. He was fluent in several languages and although he appeared to be an art lover it was a superficial love. WEN cared only for the pictures, sculptures and music he actually liked. He certainly didn't appreciate art for its own sake.

Immediately after their wedding in 1818, accompanied by a retinue of liveried servants and crates and crates of luggage, they set off on honeymoon with a string of carriages. Boarding the ferry, they crossed the English Channel to the mainland where they would travel through most of western Europe, spending a lot of time in France, Switzerland and Italy.

This was known as "The Grand Tour" and was so popular with the rich that travellers frequently met up with relatives, friends and neighbours.

Honeymoons for the privileged classes could last years. Consequently, by the time they arrived back in England, the "newlyweds" had usually acquired a family and Fanny and WEN Nightingale were no exception. Of all the countries they visited, being a cultured and sophisticated couple, they loved Italy best and spent most of their time there. And within a year of marrying, their first child was born while they were staying in Naples.

Standing at the foot of Mount Vesuvius, the port of Naples is renowned for its splendid buildings and sculptures. And because it was so beautiful, the new parents decided to give their pretty daughter its name. But charming though the name was for a splendid city, Naples seemed inappropriate for a baby so they compromised and gave her its Greek name, Parthenope. Before long, this was reduced to an affectionate "Pop" and stayed thus for some time.

Two years later, they were staying in Florence where they'd rented a house, the Villa Colombaia. A long, low building with shuttered windows, well laid "Italian" gardens and a profusion of shady trees, it stood high up in the Tuscany hills overlooking the city's canals, bridges, piazzas and magnificent buildings. Here, on 12th May 1820, the Nightingales were blessed with a second daughter. This time they chose Florence for the child's name. That quickly turned into Flo.

Even now the name Parthenope is unknown for a girl, but in that day, so was Florence. Indeed, it is claimed the Nightingales' daughter was the first ever to bear the name.

After a further year touring, when Pop was aged three and Flo one, WEN and Fanny declared it was time they returned and settled in their newly-built home in Derbyshire in the north of England.

Architecturally designed by WEN himself, Lea Hurst was a beautiful house standing on a rise in an isolated spot close to the River Derwent.

The house teemed with servants and nurse-maids. It had fifteen bedrooms, a sumptuous drawing-room, music-room and library. Fanny had her private boudoir where she could retire for privacy or entertain special friends. WEN had a study and smoking-room for the same purpose.

Despite this luxury, until the twentieth century, nurseries tended to be purely func-tional and the Nightingales followed this trend. The children didn't even have the comfort of a carpeted floor; just a small mat. There wasn't a cushion in sight for the hard, upright chairs, and the table in the centre of the room was of unpolished whitewood. They even slept in an open bed – at a time when beds normally had curtains all round to keep out cold in the winter and flying insects in summer.

Unfortunately, beautiful though Lea Hurst was, it soon proved impractical because Fanny thought a fifteen-bedroomed home was too small and anyway, it was too far away from the social whirl she loved. Also, at a time before central heating when people relied on coal or wood fires burning in the hearth, it was impossible to keep the building warm in winter when howling winds blew across the land.

After four years, in 1825, when Pop was seven and Flo five, planning to use Lea Hurst only in the spring and autumn, the family moved to Hampshire in the south of England and made their main home in a much larger place. Redbrick Embley House, situated on the edge of the New Forest, had further advantages as their dearest friends, the Palmerstons, lived close by – Viscount Henry Palmerston was then Secretary of State for War.

PAM, as he was called, could be a bit boorish and brusque. Unless they knew him well, people tended not to like him. Children found him quite intimidating, but Flo was always fond of him, and of all the homes she visited she particularly liked his home, Broadlands.

11

They had relatives living close by as well, the Bonham-Carters, whose daughter Hilary was one of Flo's favourite cousins.

Like most people of their station, the Nightingales stayed in London during the "Season": May, June and July when everybody attended balls, garden parties, regattas, Ascot races, and the opera and rode in Rotten Row each day.

Late summer and early autumn saw entire households moving north for the grouse shooting or, as in the Nightingales' case, to Derbyshire for the partridge shoot and fox and stag hunting, followed by a grand Hunt Ball. Then, with the onset of winter, they were on the move south again to their Hampshire home, Embley Park.

WEN had brothers and sisters and Fanny was one of ten children, so Flo and Pop had lots of aunts and uncles with numerous children of their own. This meant the girls were never without young companions because they were always either visiting or being visited by them.

Of all the children in this extended family, Flo stood out as being somehow a bit odd and was often quite serious. She liked playing with toys and joined in all the games but she didn't seem to enjoy them as much as the rest did. She liked reading, though, and she was an ardent music lover. Some of her happiest hours were spent playing piano duets with her precocious cousin,

Marianne Nicholson, who was as keen on music as she was.

If a family pet or any animal on the estate was sick or injured, Flo gave it her undivided attention until it was nursed back to health. And the favourite kind of visitors to her home were those with babies. Then she could disappear into the austere nursery and help take care of them.

While she was doing this or nursing her sick or wounded pets, broken or damaged dolls and toy animals, everybody smiled indulgently and spoke among themselves of her tender nature and kindness. Little did anyone suspect that in future years, those tendencies would cause much heartache – and merit great honour.

Flo was only six when she too began to realize how different she was from others. It started when she first became aware of what futile lives the women in her social sphere were expected to lead – and that the same fate awaited her. Still, other girls happily accepted this, so she thought there was something seriously wrong with her mind.

Her mother and father were worried, too, and confided to relatives that they believed they'd "hatched a wild swan". Flo had such fluctuating moods. One hour she could be overcome with shyness and retreat into a quiet corner. The next, with the flimsiest excuse, she was flying into a raving tantrum.

The two sisters spent their earliest years in the school-room with a stream of governesses. None of them stayed long because they couldn't tolerate Fanny's interference. WEN was sick and tired of their constant comings and goings, so when Parthe – she'd outgrown Pop – was aged fourteen and Flo twelve, he took over their education.

He taught them history, philosophy and mathematics plus Greek, Latin, French, German and Italian. This was most unusual in an age when education was only deemed necessary for boys.

WEN was especially fluent in Italian but, as with his dilettante love of art, he spoke it like a native rather than as a scholar, paying little attention to grammar. Florence, on the other hand, was pedantic, and gave particular attention to that branch of all five languages she was learning.

She took all her education seriously, delighting in mathematics and world history, while her sister merely studied them out of duty.

Fanny, being of a different nature, was more concerned with social status. Her single goal was to be an outstanding figure in fashionable society and she expected her daughters to follow her example.

14

Women were expected to look pale and to be frail, weepy, demure and given to frequent attacks of the vapours – fainting. They were to develop such skills as painting, singing, dancing, playing musical instruments and doing intricate needlework like petit-point and lace-making. Preoccupied with their appearance, they spent hours fretting about their hair, complexions, clothes and jewellery, and practising social graces.

The only practical achievement expected was the ability to manage domestic staff because a woman's ultimate fulfilment was in making a good marriage, though not necessarily a loving one.

Though Flo shared her mother's great beauty, to Fanny's consternation she didn't have any of these aspirations. On the contrary, regarding her personal aims, she seemed to have more of the Smith male interests.

Fanny's family were very politically motivated. From 1753 to 1785, Samuel, her grandfather, had blatantly supported the Americans in their War of Independence against Britain. Her own father was an active opponent of slavery and a long-time devotee of William Wilberforce.

Fanny was delighted with her older daughter, though, as Pop appeared to be growing up to be the epitome of sweet, demure womanhood.

Sadly, though, while conforming to all her mother's interests, she lacked her grace, beauty and wit.

She always felt inferior to Florence and bitterly resented her beauty and brains, yet at the same time she was possessive of her, demanding all her time and devotion.

Still, Parthe had the edge when it came to artistic talent. She did all the flower arranging in the house and, although her sketchings were really no more than a fruitless pastime, they were worthy of exhibition. That, of course, could never have been considered for it too was a male preserve.

So, while Parthe was learning to assume her correct role in society, her sister was inwardly rebelling against it. Outside the confining grandeur of their homes was a world full of interest and excitement. Above all, there were causes to fight for. She didn't want her life to be an endless succession of house-parties, picnics, balls and holidays.

It wasn't that Flo didn't approve of all these activities along with visits to and from friends and relatives and the constant preparations for family celebrations – comings of age, engagements, weddings and christenings. Happily, there were few funerals as the family was blessed with longevity.

As for wearing fabulous jewellery, buying

clothes, trying the latest hair fashions and learning the newest dances, well, she was maturing into a beautiful young woman who took a pride in her appearance, so she thoroughly enjoyed it all.

What made her restive and discontented was knowing she would never be allowed to do anything else. Her life was similar to an everlasting Christmas. No matter how enjoyable the festive season is, if we didn't soon return to normal, everyday life, the excitement would soon fade into boredom. And there would be nothing to look forward to.

Fanny and Parthe believed they did return to normal after such revelries. But normality to them meant taking up their embroidery, writing copious "thank you" letters to their most recent hostesses, walking in the garden or choosing and being fitted for new clothes to wear at the next grand occasion.

The closest Fanny Nightingale came to actual employment was approving the day's menus – already compiled for her by the cook. Fanny never set foot in the kitchen and had no idea how to boil an egg, let alone prepare a family meal. She didn't even run her own bathwater.

Visiting other people's homes did relieve the monotony a little for Florence, but there the conversation would be of feminine trivia while the men were engaged in serious talk. As she got older, how she longed to join them, discussing the national economy, trade, education, even crime and punishment and what had been said by whom in the House of Commons that week.

But politics, economics and social problems were strictly male preserves. Intelligence in women, particularly very young ladies not yet "come out" into society, was considered unfeminine and not to be encouraged. All the knowledge her father had imparted to her in the schoolroom was bubbling over, aching to be made use of. But all she was expected to do was indulge in idle chit-chat and useless pursuits.

This inner turmoil began to make Flo think she was completely mad. Why, she wondered, did she long to go to university like her male cousins when their sisters and her own sister, Parthe, would have fainted at the very prospect?

Self-doubt haunted her every waking hour and was manifested in the strangest ways. So convinced was she that there was something very wrong with her mind, she grew afraid of speaking to people in case she said something stupid.

When she and Parthe were old enough to leave the nursery for meals, if they were attending something grand such as a wedding breakfast and Flo was faced with an impressive table setting, she had a horror of picking up the wrong knife, fork or spoon. To overcome this

18

she perfected a delay whereby she waited until others began the meal and watched closely to ensure she followed them correctly.

She began taking refuge in "dreams" in which she could mentally absent herself from company and the silly gossip going on around her.

Another means of venting her frustrations and holding on to her sanity was by committing her thoughts to paper. She wrote hundreds of little notes.

As the years went by, while outwardly playing a passive role to please her mother, Flo sensed that a powerful and dominant personality was gradually developing under the act. But in her environment, she wondered whatever would be the use of her growing strength of character.

Then at Embley Park – on 7th February 1837, as she wrote in her diary – when she was just four months short of her seventeenth birthday, Flo heard God speaking to her, directing her on a mission. But He didn't make clear what He actually wanted her to do.

2.

THE DEBUTANTES

Florence was convinced she'd heard the Lord call her to serve Him, and she added this to her other worries. For hours she lay awake at night wondering what form that service would take. Whatever it was, she prayed it would help her escape from her pointless existence and empty future. Every day she waited for the call to be repeated, but it wasn't.

As weeks went by disillusionment set in and she grew desperate. Had she imagined it in one of her dreams? she asked herself. If God hadn't really spoken to her and there was no escape, then only death seemed attractive. But surely, she reasoned, if I really did hear Him, wishing for death will render me unworthy to serve Him. With that she resigned herself to being patient, but it wasn't until many months later when, it seemed, the answer was revealed.

As the constant social whirl continued, all the cousins who had played together as children were growing into young men and women. And among these was John Smithurst.

He was a few years older than Florence and all through their lives they'd spent a lot of time together, at Lea Hurst, at his own home nearby and at various family house-parties. But now they were grown up, their feelings towards each other began to change, and at seventeen Florence soon realised she and John were in love.

At last, God had given a clear indication of how He wanted her to serve Him. John was an ordained minister of the church so what better way than to marry one of the Lord's dedicated servants? Suddenly, for the first time in her life, the prospect of marriage, children and home-making became so important they were all she cared about.

To her horror, though, both their families were bitterly opposed to their relationship and forbade John and Flo ever to meet again.

The Smithursts didn't relish the idea of their son marrying a first cousin, let alone this strange niece of theirs.

The Nightingales felt the same about the first cousins marrying but even if they hadn't been related, they hoped she would make a better match.

John Smithurst was only a simple young curate. With his background they knew he could rise to greater heights – bishop or even arch-bishop – but that would be many years hence.

In two years' time Flo was being presented

at Court for her "coming out". She would be meeting the most eligible men in the land – royalty even. And even putting such aspirations aside, with her beauty and brains she could marry a man of vast fortune or someone with a promising career, maybe in politics. The Nightingales – and Fanny in particular – were adamant she shouldn't settle for anything less. Love was the last reason for people to marry. Only money and status counted.

There was nothing Flo could do and John Smithurst was heartbroken. A month later he left England for the desolate wilds of Canada, declaring that he would spend the rest of his life there, ministering to the Eskimos.

Flo was desperately unhappy too and she was more puzzled than ever about her call from the Lord. She'd been so confident He'd wanted her to spend her life at John's side. So what did He want of her?

Now her beloved John was forever lost to the Inuits of the frozen wastes, once more she retreated into her "dreams" and lost all interest in marriage prospects.

Ironically, young men found her the more attractive of the two sisters. This gave rise to further resentment, especially when Parthe was intent on the life destined by her position, to find a socially suitable and wealthy husband.

For some time WEN and Fanny had been

thinking of taking their daughters to the continent and now seemed the best time for a number of reasons. It would launch them into adult society abroad and provide valuable experience in preparation for their "coming out" within the next two years. It would heal the breach caused by the matter of John and Flo, and it would also be the last opportunity for them all to take a lengthy holiday together. Once the girls "came out" they would probably be betrothed or married before the "Season" was over.

Being young and having been happy with John for only a very short time, Florence recovered quickly from her lost love and was ecstatic at the prospect of the Grand Tour – her first visit abroad.

It was September, 1837, when they set off in a splendid carriage that had been built specifically to William's plans. Its three pairs of horses boasted two colourful liveried postillions. At the rear, six servants travelled with the luggage in a string of less ostentatious coaches, making up an even longer procession than on the honeymoon.

After Florence discovered she wasn't a good sailor, they landed in France from where they made a leisurely journey south to Italy.

When she was only moving from one part of England to another, Flo had always preferred arriving to travelling because it bored her. By way of diversion on this protracted journey, she planned to keep records of distances travelled each day and how long it took.

She kept meticulous lists of departure and arrival times and of all problems encountered on the way. Every physical detail of each place they stayed at, or merely passed through, was written down. She also took the trouble to discover its particular culture and customs, its social conditions, the living standards of the peasant, middle and upper classes, the laws and bye laws. Everything of the slightest interest was methodically entered in her journal.

They spent Christmas in Nice, then journeyed on to Italy where the girls were entranced by its vivid blue skies, olive groves and vineyards.

In Florence, they visited the cathedral, Giotto's belltower and Palazzo Vecchio. Flo was taken to her birthplace, Villa Colombaia, and stood in the drawing-room on the very spot where she had been baptised.

By springtime it was on to Naples to show Parthenope her birthplace and to view the early Christian paintings on catacomb walls.

Through friends, they were invited to lots of social functions where they were introduced to foreign royalty and aristocracy, revolutionaries and anarchists. It was all very exciting with its mixed elements of grandeur, daring and danger.

Flo felt deeply for the rebels fighting to free Italy from Austrian rule. They seemed to match her own inner fight for freedom.

In Rome they gazed in awe at statues and arches, at the Colosseum, the Forum, Michelangelo's Sistine Chapel ceiling, and they walked along the Appian Way.

From Italy they journeyed on to Switzerland where most of the holiday was spent at Geneva beside the lake, then to France and Paris, staying in the fashionable Place Vendome.

Here they met Mary Clarke, a well-known socialite who became a lifelong friend, known to the Nightingale family as "Clarkey".

As in every other place they visited, there was so much to do and see in Paris: Notre Dame, Sacre Coeur, and the Champs-Elysées with its newly erected Arc de Triomphe.

They walked beside the Seine and visited museums, art galleries and theatres. Clarkey took them to balls and banquets. They attended soirées at her home where they met painters, writers and, best of all for Flo, musicians. She revelled in a round of operas and concerts, awarding each one marks for merit.

Completely immersed in the gaiety and activity, not once on the tour did Florence display any of her old melancholy and Fanny was delighted. At last, it seemed, she'd come to her senses and adjusted to her correct role in life.

In the spring of 1839, however, as their Grand Tour was nearing its end, Flo was suddenly conscious that in those two years she'd heard no further call from God. Indeed, along with her love for John Smithurst, the memory of it had been chased from her mind. She hadn't even recalled it while she was standing on the steps of the greatest church in the world, St Peter's Basilica in Rome.

She was racked with guilt at her irresponsible behaviour. How could I expect to be called when every minute has been consumed with pleasure seeking? she chided herself. Now more than ever she'd proved herself unworthy and was completely discredited.

But perhaps, she thought, if from now on I put my mind to attaining worthiness, if I devote every moment preparing for it, God may call me again.

They were home at Embley Park in the April but two weeks later moved on to Lea Hurst, where Flo celebrated her nineteenth birthday. And what with her birthday and the excitement of her imminent "coming out", Flo's good intentions were quickly forgotten again.

Two weeks after her birthday in May they were all in London for the Season. Every day there were garden-parties, riding in Rotten Row and strolling in Cremorne Gardens, Chelsea. Evenings were filled with balls, theatre visits, operas and dinner-parties.

In between those activities, all the energies and interests of Fanny, Parthe and Florence were directed towards the "coming out".

As debutantes 1839 was, in effect, *their* year. Parties and balls were held solely in the girls' honour, which cost their father a colossal amount of money. And for all the different occasions, that year especially, a lot of time went into choosing and having fittings for splendid gowns of tulle, satin and taffeta, with silk for Ascot and frothy cottons for the Henley Regatta.

For the presentation to Queen Victoria at the Royal Court they would wear white diaphanous dresses – bought while they were in Paris – and long white gloves.

All the debutantes spent hours practising their curtseys for the presentation to the Queen and also for Queen Charlotte's ball at St James's Palace.

In the late eighteenth century when George III was on the throne, to celebrate his wife Charlotte's birthday, a huge edifice of a cake, weighing all of 500lbs and topped by lighted candles, was drawn into the room by maids of honour. All the women in the room had curtseyed to it and established an annual tradition for the London Season.

Accompanied by nine beats of a drum, all the debutantes would curtsey to the cake. Beginning to go down on the first beat, they must stay down with head bowed for five beats then slowly rise again. During rehearsals everybody kept wobbling and giggling and it took ages to perfect.

The girls were "coming out" at the same time as their cousin, Marianne Nicholson. The Nicholsons lived at Waverley Abbey at Farnham in Surrey but when in London for the Season they stayed at the same hotel as the Nightingales.

As children, although they had little in common except their love of music, Flo had always been very fond of Marianne. Now she had grown into a beautiful young woman with a sharp wit, charm and slight air of insolence, Flo was captivated by her. Sadly, Marianne didn't care very much for her – but her brother, Henry, did.

As with John Smithurst, the cousins had spent a lot of time in each other's company when they were children but they hadn't met since the Nightingales went to Europe.

In that time, like his sister, Flo had blossomed into a lovely young lady. She was of average height, slender and so graceful her walk was almost a glide. She had luxuriant chestnut hair. Her grey eyes danced. Her deep voice was soft and warm and Henry Nicholson soon came to adore her.

While Flo basked in Marianne's presence, Henry danced attendance on her without her noticing. She accepted all his theatre and dinner invitations but that was because her idol, Marianne, was going too. It never occurred to her that he was in love with her. Henry was simply one of the family.

Both families were aware of his feelings though, and the Nicholsons didn't have the same reservations as the Smithursts and Nightingales over first cousins marrying. Still, WEN and Fanny weren't too worried about the relationship. Henry was very young and as he was due to start at Cambridge University in the autumn, they hoped it was just a boyish infatuation that would fade once he got involved in his studies.

Henry wasn't the only one to fall in love with Florence and this struck a sour note with Parthenope. She was the one who sought attention, yet it was her sister who attracted all the young men. It was always Flo they flocked to immediately she entered a ballroom. It was Flo's dance card that was soon filled up while Parthe's was made up with the names of those left over.

Throughout that summer, Flo suffered a terrible inner conflict. She was having a wonderful time, yet in her quieter moments she expected to hear God call her again – but the voice didn't speak.

At the end of the Season, the family travelled north to Lea Hurst for the shooting and hunting.

The hectic social round continued but everything seemed an anti-climax after the excitement of the Grand Tour and the "coming out".

Over the next couple of years, Fanny continued introducing potential husbands to her daughters. To Parthe's consternation it was still Flo the young men pursued. Hoping to secure a well connected wife for their sons, ambitious mothers preyed on her, too.

All this annoyed Florence so much that Fanny worried that her erratic moods and her "dreaming" might return. When Florence was twenty-one, her mother suggested it was time she started accompanying Parthe and herself on their charitable missions, doing "lady's work".

This disgusted Florence. While it involved visiting the sick or the poor, only infection-free houses might be entered. "Ladies" shouldn't venture where they could fall victims to disease.

The previous summer had seen the poorest harvest in years and there was danger of famine spreading throughout the area with all its attendant misery and sickness. But these "ladies" considered it enough to dole out useless advice along with bowls of soup, bread and a few coins when Flo knew where the real need lay.

If a mother lay sick, with her children hungry and her husband out trying to find work, she needed someone to cook and clean for them and help nurse her. But that wouldn't be considered correct behaviour so the "ladies" walked on to the next house.

Reluctantly, Flo obeyed her mother. She and Parthe demurely walked behind her through the village and along the lanes while Fanny pointed out certain cottages and houses where it would be unwise to venture. Flo would clench her fists, digging her nails into her palms while forcing herself to obey when all the time she longed to break free and go where she could do some real good.

One evening in the summer of 1842, at a dinner party at the home of Lord Palmerston – PAM's – Flo was introduced to Richard Monckton Milnes. She was twenty-two at the time. He was thirty-three, eleven years her senior.

She already knew something about him. He was a Member of Parliament, rich, well travelled, a poet and, like herself, an accomplished linguist and music lover. He lived in Pall Mall in London and was noted for his breakfast parties at which, among many other notable people, he entertained such distinguished literary figures as William Thackeray, Alfred Lord Tennyson and Thomas Carlyle.

What Florence hadn't been told about Richard was how extremely handsome he was with laughing grey eyes, golden hair and a sparkling wit that kept her laughing throughout the evening.

Also at the dinner-party was Richard's friend, the eminent German scientist Baron Robert Wilhelm Bunsen, who was convalescing in England after losing an eye in a laboratory experiment. And both men were about to make an enormous impact on Florence's life.

3.

INFLUENTIAL ENCOUNTERS

When the men left the dinner-table to join the ladies in the drawing-room, the Baron wandered over to the group Flo was in. In the ensuing conversation, the word Kaiserworth kept being mentioned. Everybody but Flo seemed to know what he was talking about so she pressed him for an explanation.

The Kaiserworth Institute in Germany had been founded sixteen years earlier by a young Lutheran cleric, Theodor Fliendner, and his wife. To begin with they'd converted their summer home into a hostel for discharged prisoners. Later, in 1836, they'd extended the building to accommodate an orphanage, a mental asylum, a detention centre for young offenders, a teacher training school and a hospital where women were trained in nursing.

All over the world, nurses had notorious reputations but at Kaiserworth only respectable widows or unmarried girls with no marriage prospects were accepted. Their training also included cooking, laundry and gardening. They received religious instruction and were taught how to counsel the bereaved. They frequently tended patients in their own homes and provided for the destitute out of the Institute's funds. Theodor and his wife had recently published a book about the Institute which doubled as a textbook for nursing.

Eminent people went to see for themselves how the place was run and Elizabeth Fry, the renowned prison reformer, had been so impressed when she visited it, she was considering founding a nursing order herself.

Flo was fascinated and as Baron Bunsen continued she felt a stirring in her heart.

She recalled the childhood pleasures of tending visitors' babies in the nursery, of nursing broken dolls and sick animals. What satisfaction there would be in learning how to really nurse and help heal humans, she thought.

This was when she got the first real inkling of what she wanted to do with her life.

As for the other man she met that night, it was quite obvious to everybody that Flo and Richard were very attracted to each other. And to her family's delight he began a serious courtship which Flo clearly welcomed.

Her cousin, young Henry Nicholson, also continued paying court to her so WEN and Fanny were pleased that someone else had come into her life. Flo's future seemed settled.

Apart from all Richard's flattering attention, Flo's life continued much as usual with her daily activities consisting of reading, writing letters, playing the piano and taking charge of the linen cupboard.

Fanny and WEN were very interested in reforms of every kind and in June 1844, when Flo was aged twenty-four, they invited Dr Samuel Gridley Howe and his wife to stay at Embley Park.

Dr Howe was a famous American philanthropist. He devoted his life to helping others and had recently been offered the post of Director at a newly established Institute for the Blind in Boston, Massachusetts.

Before committing himself, though, he needed to gain some idea of what it meant to be blind, so he spent an entire week blindfolded. At the end of the trial he was grazed and black and blue from bumping into furniture and tripping over things.

Now he was touring Europe, studying advanced teaching methods for the blind and enrolling tutors for the Perkins Institute in Boston.

Flo knew that being of liberal mind and an American, he wasn't preoccupied with convention. So one evening at dinner, she drew gasps of horror by suddenly asking if he thought it would be unsuitable and dishonourable if she were to become a nurse in a hospital. "Would it be a dreadful thing to do?" she asked.

Dr Howe admired a strong-minded woman. His wife, Julia, was a prime example of one for she'd composed America's Battle Hymn of the Republic. That had endeared her to Fanny's family being keen supporters of the War of Independence. But they soon became disappointed in her husband.

Without hesitation, the eminent man considered Flo's an excellent idea and advised her, "Go ahead. Do whatever you think is right for you, and God bless you".

Flo's parents and Parthe were stunned to silence that a guest in their house should be so disrespectful and give her such unsound advice.

At that time, only nuns were considered suitable for nursing because secular nurses were of the very lowest social class – drunken, immoral, criminal. And anyway, *ladies* didn't *earn* a living. Working for payment was strictly for lower-class women.

But with Dr Howe's endorsement, nursing as a vocation became even more attractive and after his visit ended, Flo begged to be allowed to go and study the techniques at Salisbury Infirmary.

She planned to learn all she could, then return to Embley Park and set up a nurse training establishment nearby. It would be a non-religious order where respectable, intelligent women would be trained, not only in nursing, but more importantly, in nurse training. From there the scheme would snowball when the qualified nurse tutors set up their own training establishments.

But when her parents heard these plans they strictly forbade it. In a way, they had good reason.

Apart from nurses' low moral standards, hospitals were undesirable places in themselves. In the days leading up to the discovery of anaesthetics and antiseptics, they were filthy, germ-ridden havens of disease that echoed to the groans and screams of the suffering.

Rich people could afford to be attended in their own homes by nuns or private nurses; yet even these were ignorant of proper skills and quite unable to combat the spread of disease, as germs hadn't yet been discovered.

Nevertheless, at least Flo fully understood what she wanted to do. She also knew she would never be permitted to do it and she became very depressed, moping about all the time.

Her favourite aunt, Mai Smith, was William's sister, married to Fanny's brother, Sam. This made her Flo's closest aunt and she was the only person she could turn to.

Mai Smith was fully occupied with caring for her family but being of a rather independent nature she understood how Flo felt. She had seen numbers of intelligent women succumb to breakdowns when every little problem was blown into a crisis in their empty minds. Some actually went insane and all because of the idleness thrust upon them by social convention.

To keep her niece from retreating into that sort of mental cocoon, Mai asked her to concentrate on finding a subject for studying that the family *would* approve.

Flo pondered a while. She was already fluent in several languages and she was well read. At last she decided mathematics might benefit her.

At this, Mai approached Fanny suggesting that Flo should take up some pastime of academic interest to get her out of her depression, adding, diplomatically, that it would be useful to her when she was married. What did she think about a course in mathematics? They could engage a good-living, elderly, married man to tutor her on a three-year course.

Fanny grudgingly agreed to it all. Two lessons a week with two hours of study each day were arranged, but they were to be given at her uncle Octavius's house – another of Fanny's brothers. In return Flo would act as companion to his young children.

Eagerly Flo embarked on her tuition and aunt Mai, who was staying there at the time, got up at six with her every morning and lit a fire in the library so she could get on with the work before the rest of the household was astir.

Then after only one month, Fanny stopped the lessons saying they were keeping Flo from her duties at home. Despite this setback Flo had learned an inordinate amount and was particularly interested in compiling statistics and making graphs.

On returning home, unknown to anyone, she continued her studies in her room, still getting up at dawn.

That Christmas was spent at the Nicholsons' home, Waverley Abbey, where everybody had a wonderful time with a masked ball. Flo stage-managed a production of *The Merchant of Venice* in which various family members took roles. And yet there were times when she felt she simply couldn't go downstairs and join in the festivities. What would face her after they were over and she was left in the mental vacuum of "passing the time away"?

There was something else to contemplate on during that Christmas time. Although everyone else had known it all the time, she discovered Henry was in love with her and he asked her to marry him. She was so shocked and tongue-tied, her mumbled response gave the impression she needed time to think.

Over the past five years, Henry had graduated from Cambridge and had been working hard to forge a secure position in the world, one that would enable him to afford to marry.

Ever since her parents had broken up her relationship with John Smithurst, Flo had never contemplated marriage. She was in love with Richard Monckton but she was still waiting for that call from God, confident it would come one day.

When the family were returning home to Embley, Henry's younger brother, William, asked to go with them. His parents agreed but when they asked why, Parthe told them she believed it was because Flo had been coaching him in mathematics and he wanted to continue until it was time to return to Sandhurst Military Academy. At this his father exploded. A *girl* coaching his son. If that got out, he would be the laughing stock of the Academy. He would be disgraced and might even have to leave.

Fanny and WEN made profuse apologies and left. But after they were back at Embley Park they kept on writing their apologies and there was a coolness between the two families for quite a while.

A year went by during which they'd grown friendly again. Then in 1845, when Henry was aged twenty-five, he again asked Flo to marry him. This time she was prepared and when she refused him, he was heartbroken and trouble erupted again.

Though she was fond of her, Henry's sister, Marianne, had always seemed awesome to Flo. Marianne worshipped her handsome brother and when Flo rejected him she was enraged.

How dare she treat him so badly after six years of courtship? she demanded to know. She accused Flo of flirting, teasing and leading him to believe she loved him and she vowed never to speak to her again. The whole incident created another rift between the two families.

Flo was so upset at the whole incident and especially at losing Marianne's valued friendship that she retreated into her old "dreams" as she called them.

She took stock of the past eight years she'd spent waiting for a second call from the Lord and she looked ahead at an even bleaker, emptier future because the call hadn't come.

William and Fanny knew she was in love with Richard Monckton and that he'd proposed to her more than once and she'd refused him. Now Fanny asked Flo how long she intended keeping him waiting. When Flo replied that she didn't want to marry him, her mother was furious, rebuking her for forsaking her duty to her father. How much longer did she expect him to keep her?

But what of her duty to God and to her own inner feelings? Flo asked herself. Even if she wasn't yet worthy to serve Him, she'd heard

41

His call. To remind herself it wasn't all a dream she would open her diary and look at the date where she'd written: "God spoke and called me to His service". To go against what she knew was true would be spiritual suicide, she decided, so she would go on waiting.

Elizabeth Gaskell, the famous author of the books *Cranford* and *Mary Barton*, was a friend of the Nightingales and often visited them, especially when they were at Lea Hurst, as she lived in the next county, Cheshire.

She noticed during one of her stays that Flo was often late for meals with excuses that she'd been doing "ladies' work". Elizabeth thought this strange as it was something she'd always objected to and undertaken with great reluctance.

Then one day she came across her sitting in the garden, writing a letter to her cousin Hilary and looking very sad. Elizabeth sat beside her and encouraged her to tell her what was wrong.

Flo had been doing "ladies work" but not the sort her mother approved of. She'd been going into houses where she was truly needed, rolling up her sleeves and getting down to work, cleaning, washing dishes and preparing meals.

But that morning, utterly helpless, she'd stood at a bedside and watched a young woman die. Some people were supposed to have been caring for her, but they hadn't *nursed* her at all. They simply sat there, watching her, talking amongst themselves and giving her the occasional drink.

Flo faced the fact that if she'd had nursing experience the woman might still have died, but at least she could have made some effort to save her. At the very least she could have eased the way to her inevitable death. But, she told Elizabeth, she'd felt like a spectator, standing there, completely ignorant of all medical knowledge.

In the summer of 1846 while they were in London for the Season, Baron Bunsen lent her the book that Theodor Fliendner had written, *The Year Book of the Institution of Protestant Deaconesses at Kaiserworth in Germany*.

Flo was so fascinated by the title she took the trouble to find out what exactly deaconesses were and discovered the word is taken from the Greek language and means "to serve". The first recorded deaconess was Phoebe who had tended St Paul and was later assigned to take his letter to the Romans.

Before that, nursing was the duty of slaves but even they were never trained to tend the sick. They merely kept them clean and fed them.

After reading the book, Flo pointed all this out to her parents and sister. They couldn't dispute that the Deaconesses were reputable *and* they were nursing. Still they insisted it was wrong for a well brought up Victorian girl to think of such an occupation.

At thirty, she didn't need parental consent to do whatever she pleased, but going against them was something a well brought up Victorian miss couldn't consider.

Flo, in common with Fanny and Parthe, could fall "ill" any time it suited. She wasn't consciously putting on an act but genuinely believed she was ill with headaches, nausea and fainting. After reading the book she became so frustrated she was forever suffering from all three, with additional coughs and sneezes. She became more depressed than ever.

Some family friends, Charles and Selina Bracebridge, who looked on Flo as a daughter, were sure she was heading for a complete breakdown and were very worried about her. They'd planned to spend the winter in Rome so, remembering how Flo had enjoyed the Grand Tour, they asked WEN and Fanny if they could take her with them.

As was the norm while touring on the Continent, they bumped into lots of people they knew. One day while standing on the steps of St Peter's Basilica, Charles and Selina introduced Flo to Sidney Herbert. He was a half-brother to the Earl of Pembroke and a very wealthy man, a devout Christian and philanthropist whose generosity to tenants on his estates was well known. A Member of Parliament, he had been Foreign Secretary in Sir Robert Peel's government but was now out of office. When they met he was in Rome on honeymoon with his beautiful young wife, Elizabeth.

They all spent the rest of the holiday together during which the Herberts and Flo became firm friends. Like the Bracebridges, Sidney and Liz were modern in their outlook and could see nothing wrong in wanting to be a nurse. They themselves took a lot of interest in health care.

One day they all went to a convent school, the Trinita de Monti, which was known for its innovative teaching methods. It was the Bracebridges who wanted to know how the system worked. But Flo was so impressed it crossed her mind that if nursing was always going to be taboo, she might consider teaching and set up a little school somewhere. That wouldn't cause any dispute. Lots of people in her social circle ran schools for the poor. It was a form of "lady's work".

Those encounters with both the Herberts and the nuns in the convent school encouraged Flo to have more confidence in herself and she determined to take more control over her own life in the future.

But as soon as she was back home after six months' absence, her mother ordered her to make an inventory of all the household effects:

linen, silverware, crockery, ornaments and larder stores. Flo felt she was imprisoned again. While making list after list, she made her mind up. As soon as the inventory was completed she would tell her family she intended opening a village school near Lea Hurst.

The proposition was welcomed as a splendid idea and within weeks her little academy was established.

Not all the village children attended but Flo had a fair sized class and for a time she enjoyed the work. But soon she realised that, even though it was only an elementary education she was giving, teaching like nursing could only be successfully done if the teacher had been properly trained and Flo hadn't. Much as she loved children, she had to admit that general education wasn't her forte while nursing was in her blood.

Her mother and Parthe had changed their minds, too. They started reprimanding her for spending so much time away from home when she should be keeping them company. She'd already spent the winter gadding about Europe. Her school couldn't have stayed open long anyway. It was nearly the end of autumn. The family would soon move south for the winter and Lea Hurst would be closed down.

4.

FREEDOM

Back in Embley Park for the winter, Florence resumed her secret mathematical studies and wrote copious letters to friends and relatives.

From these letters, most people could deduce that she was in a poor mental state, so steeped in self-pity as to be bordering on the paranoid.

Clarkey, now Mrs Julius Mohle and living in Germany, contacted Baron Bunsen and suggested they should do something to help her. Other friends and acquaintances rallied round. They knew where her interests lay and everybody began gathering all the information available on hospitals and nursing and sent the papers to Florence.

Each day at dawn, before the servants came to open the curtains and rouse her, she got up and spent two hours studying hospital management and annual reports. But these were all "official" documents and some were grossly out of date. Flo sensed there was much they didn't tell her – and she was right.

In the days before anaesthetics were discovered, the only means of easing pain – particularly under the torture of surgery – was by giving patients alcohol or dangerous drugs such as opium or laudanum.

They were all potential killers. Alcohol accelerated the blood flow so patients often bled to death. And when someone was treated over a long period for a painful complaint they became either alcoholics or drug addicts. If they didn't die from the complaint, their analgesic killed them anyway.

Hospitals were so awful that people were terrified of going, especially if it was for an operation. If they were strong enough they literally fought off anybody trying to take them there. Patients knew, whether they were young or old, that not many left hospital alive. Expectant mothers usually lost their babies at birth and only a few of the mothers themselves survived.

In the majority of cases, it was through a lack of simple hygiene. Doctors and nurses would deliver a baby to one mother then, without so much as washing their hands, go straight to another patient who perhaps had a contagious disease.

Festering sores were dressed and then, after handling the filthy bandages, nurses would go directly to a patient who had had an amputation or an appendix removed.

Knives were never washed. Suture needles

were used over and over again. Aprons and
overalls were stiff with dried blood. Surgeons
boasted at the state of the garments because the
more dried blood there was indicated the wearer
had performed the most operations. For a sur-
geon's overall to be able to stand up on its own
was a wonderful achievement.

Wards were filled with a terrible smell and
were so crammed there was barely enough room
between the beds for anyone to walk, let alone
tend to patients. And it was normal practice
for nurses to sleep in the beds with their
patients.

Some of these horrific facts seeped through
from the reports Florence read. She had the
sense to know that since anaesthetics had been
discovered conditions were slightly improved.
But general standards would never improve
without influential people making a stand. With
that, she added politics to her studies.

This went on for three years and all the while
Richard was paying court to her. Florence loved
him dearly but the memory of God's calling was
never out of her thoughts now.

Meanwhile, aunt Mai and uncle Octavius tried
persuading Fanny and William into letting her
go to Kaiserworth to see for herself what it was
all about. Under pressure from the Bunsens and
the Mohles as well, they finally gave in and said
she could go for a couple of weeks while they

and Parthe visited Clarkey and her new husband in Frankfurt.

Then word came of a threatened revolution in Germany. Fanny gleefully took the opportunity to abandon the whole project and announced that they would all go to take the spa waters at Malvern in Worcestershire instead.

Florence couldn't believe she'd been thwarted again. Was the Lord playing some cruel trick on her? she wondered. If so, was it for being rebellious at heart while appearing to be an obedient daughter? Could it be for telling herself she only wanted to serve Him when all the time she was so in love with Richard Monckton? All sorts of possibilities swam around in her brain.

In 1849, after knowing her for seven years, Richard proposed to her again but this time, instead of politely hinting that she needed more time, she finally said No. She could never marry, either him or anyone else.

Now, surely, that would prove to God that her intentions were genuine. He had spoken to her once. He would call her again and she would be free and ready to respond.

Her family were furious when they found out. Fanny, conveniently forgetting how old she was when she married William, reminded Florence that she was almost thirty and this was her last chance. No man would ever propose to her again.

Parthe couldn't even bring herself to speak to her sister. As long as Flo remained unmarried no one would take an interest in her. She treated her so badly Flo nearly had a breakdown because on top of all this stress was her heartache at losing Richard. She couldn't eat or sleep and grew more and more depressed with each passing day.

And then the Lord came to her rescue in an unexpected way.

The Bracebridges were going on a long holiday to Egypt and Greece in the November and knowing how much good her Roman holiday had done, they asked her to go with them.

But Florence didn't enjoy this trip. She was pining for Richard and wishing she hadn't rejected him. He was a liberal-minded man. Marrying him would have given her the freedom she needed to pursue her own interests. But then again, she reasoned, how could a married woman possibly be a hospital nurse living away from home?

They spent Christmas and the New Year in Egypt but Florence took little interest in the celebrations or in viewing the Valley of the Kings, the Pyramids or the Sphinx. She did make some attempt to study hieroglyphics which at any other time would have totally absorbed her. On this occasion she couldn't concentrate for more than a few minutes.

Her sadness and depression were affecting Charles and Selina and by March, while sailing down the Nile, they were considering cutting the holiday short.

Their next stop was at Karnak, the site of ancient Thebes, where they viewed the great Temple of Rameses and the massive ruins of the Hypostyle Hall with its breathtakingly high columns.

They walked along the avenue of sphinxes and it was here in March 1850, while sitting to rest for a while, that at last, after fourteen years, God called again to Florence. Now she knew that in refusing to marry the man she loved above all else, she'd proved herself worthy to serve the Lord.

She surprised her travelling companions by suddenly cheering up and starting to take an interest in the holiday. Greece was next on the agenda and by the time they reached Athens in May, she was her old, curious self eagerly surveying the Acropolis and Mount Olympus.

While they were gazing at the Parthenon, a baby owl fell from its nest high in the ruins and lay fluttering on the ground. Florence promptly rescued it, named it Athena and spent the rest of her tour carrying it around in her pocket.

The Bracebridges, remembering her disappointment at not going to Kaiserworth, decided to travel home through Germany and let her see the place. When it was time to leave Greece they told her their plan and Florence nearly fainted from excitement.

In Germany, tours of cathedrals, galleries and castles were forsaken in favour of visiting hospitals, orphanages and, at last, the Kaiserworth Institute of Deaconesses, where Florence stayed for two weeks.

Being a religious establishment, the Institute was run on the lines of a strict convent order. Students got up at 5 am and worked for nearly an hour until they had a ten-minute break for breakfast at 6 am. This consisted of a slice of bread and some thin porridge, then back to work.

At midday there was another ten-minute break for vegetable soup. At 3 pm, another ten minutes for a piece of bread and a cup of tea, and at 7 pm they had their final ten-minute break for more soup. Then they commenced religious studies which included reading lengthy passages from the Bible.

There seemed to be endless prayers throughout the day along with nursing studies and the undertaking of household tasks, laundry and floor-scrubbing.

Medical training was poor as tutors didn't have the essential knowledge and relied largely on herbal remedies and folklore. Standards of hygiene were atrocious but care and compassion for patients shone through all the ignorance. Children were especially cared for and had a jolly time of games, stories, singing, birthday parties and, most important of all, kisses and cuddles.

Florence was very popular with everybody there and she worked hard.

Innocently, Selina wrote to Fanny telling her how well Flo had reacted to watching an operation involving the amputation of a limb. Fanny was distraught that a daughter of hers should witness such unladylike scenes and refrained from telling Parthe lest it send her hysterical.

Florence wrote home, too, telling them what a wonderful place Kaiserworth was, but her letters went unanswered. Nevertheless, she was so impressed with the Institute that she wrote a booklet about it and intended getting it published when she got home.

At the end of the holiday, the Bracebridges delivered her back home, fitter and happier than she had been in years. But her mother and sister rounded on them, accusing them of deception. Then they turned on Florence and berated her for being disobedient.

She argued that Kaiserworth was the most respectable place anyone could enter. They already knew Elizabeth Fry herself had visited it years earlier and commended it for improving nursing standards.

But her reasoning fell on deaf ears. She was forbidden even to speak about the Institute and she must never disclose to anyone that she'd been there. If news got out of her behaviour, the disgrace would be too much to bear.

After her brief glimpse of freedom and experiencing the joy of being involved in nursing, home life was even more intolerable with Fanny and Parthe carrying on screaming confrontations with her at every opportunity.

She was ordered, "as an unmarried woman approaching middle age", to respect her duty as companion to her ageing mother and demanding sister.

In October the rift with the Nicholsons was healed when they received tragic news that Henry Nicholson had been drowned in Spain. His mother was prostrate with grief and wanted Flo near her as she was the girl he'd loved.

Marianne, newly married to a construction engineer, Captain Douglas Galton, was at Waverley, too. Now her brother was dead she was even more angry with Florence and completely ignored her throughout her stay.

Aunt Anne couldn't bring herself to go and pack his belongings at his rooms in London so Florence went with her and saw to everything. But in less than a week Fanny and Parthe were demanding that she return home to Embley Park where she was most needed. Florence begged to be allowed to stay on at Waverley and was given just two more days.

Once home again, despite their attitude towards her desire to nurse, they soon took advantage of her training. WEN was going to London for treatment at an eye clinic and Flo was told to go with him and take care of him.

If she wanted to nurse there were opportunities within the family. And for the next three years she did just that, wait for orders to nurse sick relatives. In between she spent endless, tedious days of letter writing, reading and overseeing the linen cupboard.

For hours she sat listening to the clock steadily ticking away the hours of her useless life. As months went by, death seemed the only light ahead of her. She longed to go to bed one night and never wake up. Had she heard the Lord calling her again, she wondered, or was she going mad?

It was this thought that finally made her face reason. She was a grown woman who could do as she liked with her life. It was ridiculous for someone almost thirty-one to be kept a virtual prisoner by her family. To preserve her sanity she realised she would have to get away and quickly.

Then she worried about leaving because it meant having to "take" things from the house as her personal possessions weren't truly hers.

In those days an unmarried woman belonged to her father. Married, she belonged to her husband and whatever she inherited from her father also became the property of her husband.

Only unmarried women or widows who had benefited from their father's or husband's will owned anything – and even then the legacy was usually left to a male executor.

So although Flo was, as her mother had said, "approaching middle age", she was wholly dependent on the family for food, clothes, everything.

She appealed to Cardinal Manning, later to become Archbishop of Westminster, asking him to arrange for her to visit a hospital run by the Protestant Sisters of Charity. Surely her family couldn't object to that when it had been established by Elizabeth Fry, whom they admired. But they did because Cardinal Manning's religious convictions were, at that time, hovering between the Church of England and Roman Catholicism. That didn't matter to Florence but the idea of her associating with him sent Fanny ranting again.

Nevertheless, Florence contrived a way to go and see Elizabeth Fry to tell her how she admired her and what her own ambitions were. Mrs Fry was fortunate in coming from a family which was intent on reform and had never experienced the blind prejudice Flo faced, so she sympathised with the pretty, chestnut-haired girl and gave her best wishes.

When a very old great-aunt fell ill, Florence was sent to stay with her until she died.

In February she was going with her relatives, the Bonham-Carters, to visit the Mohles, presently staying in Paris, and she intended spending some time at the House of Providence run by the Catholic Sisters of Charity. But no sooner had she got there when she was ordered home to nurse her dying grandmother who was ninety-five years old. Still, she didn't mind that. At least the old lady would receive proper care in her hands.

It was 1852, and just when she'd finally determined to escape before she really did go mad, Parthe had a mental breakdown. Florence was ordered to nurse her, seeing that it was all her fault in the first place and nursing was what she wanted to do anyway.

Characteristically, Parthe was the most demanding, selfish patient imaginable and never missed an opportunity to tell Florence she had caused her breakdown. Rather than get better, she got worse as every little thing that didn't please her sent her into hysterics.

However, as the Lord often works in mysterious ways it seemed there was a way out for Florence after all.

One day the family doctor, Sir James Clark, who was also the Queen's physician, took her to one side and told her that Parthenope would never recover while Florence lived at home. He strongly advised her to get away quickly, as much for her own welfare as her sister's.

Then he suggested Mr and Mrs Nightingale take Parthe for three months' therapy to an eminent doctor at Carlsbad in Germany. This was the very opportunity Florence had been needing.

Immediately they arrived at the clinic she announced that while Parthe was having her treatment she would go and stay at the Kaiserworth Institute.

This invited more awful rows. Fanny shouted and waved her arms about wildly.

William quietly slipped away to hide.

Parthe flew into a screaming, hysterical tantrum and ended by throwing all her jewellery at Florence, hitting her full in the face. At this Flo, under all the intense pressure of the past months, fell into a dead faint.

When she came round, she calmly began packing and the following morning she finally claimed her independence and walked out, heading for Kaiserworth, where she stayed for three months.

Parthe made a remarkable recovery from her breakdown once Flo had left so the family returned home, making up all sorts of excuses for Flo's absence.

Three months' later, when she arrived home from Kaiserworth, William dreaded a resurgence of the screaming arguments, but he was mistaken. Her mother and sister wouldn't even speak to her.

5.

THE SUPERINTENDENT

Early that summer, just before the family was due to go to London for the Season, Liz Herbert was staying at Embley Park and she told Florence about the Institute for the Care of Sick Gentlewomen in London.

It was moving into a bigger building, currently being converted in Harley Street, and she'd heard they had a vacancy for a Superintendent. As Florence had done some preliminary training in Germany and had experience of nursing her sick family, why didn't she apply for the post?

Fanny was distraught when she heard this and she and Parthe soon started talking again to Florence. What would people think if she consented to stoop to such a deplorable level? Kaiserworth at least had a religious background. More importantly, it was situated abroad and not many people had found out about her being there. But Superintendent of an Institute *in London* – that couldn't be kept quiet for long.

What was worse, even though Liz had said the post didn't carry a salary, she would actually be *employed*. Had she no consideration for her family's standing in the community? Hadn't she brought enough disgrace on the Nightingale name already?

Patiently, Florence tried to explain. The Institute was a charitable organisation for 'gentlewomen' and the committee was chaired by Lady Canning, widow of a former Prime Minister, no less. Didn't her mother realize, over the past four or five years lots of notable people had begun taking interest in health care? Nursing was rapidly becoming respectable and her consideration was for the sick rather than the silly prejudices of certain people.

Naturally, this provoked more rows and raised voices echoed through the great house.

Embarrassed servants scurried behind the green baize door to their downstairs refuge.

William sought cover in the garden or his study. Eventually he moved right out and went to London, living at his gentlemen's club, the Athenaeum. From there he wrote to Parthe begging her to stop interfering in her sister's life and making their home so unhappy. He didn't dare reproach his wife, although she was equally to blame.

However, Florence applied for and was offered the post. But because she was so young

– at thirty-three – she would have to take an elderly lady of good reputation with her to act as housekeeper-cum-chaperone.

William had always been tolerant of his younger daughter's ambitious nature but he wished she'd chosen something less controversial. All the same, he was half looking forward to her departure if it meant peace would return to the house.

Florence wouldn't get a salary because nursing "gentlewomen" was considered a privilege and didn't merit financial reward, so her father granted her an annual allowance of £500. As the annual income for a similar post at that time was £10 he was being extremely generous.

Once again, her mother and sister were faced with explaining her fall from grace to all who discovered their awful secret. They didn't know she was planning – albeit anonymously – to have her booklet about Kaiserworth published.

When Florence arrived at the Institute on 12th August, 1853, she was utterly dismayed.

Builders and craftsmen were still at work renovating the place and she was expected to supervise them. There was no furniture, no carpets, curtains or bed linen. The kitchen was bare of utensils and she was given ten days to have everything organized before the first patients arrived.

She soon discovered that even when the Institute was completed there would be a terrible lack of facilities.

There would be no hot water. No means of bed-bound patients calling for help. The kitchens were so far from the wards, food would be cold by the time it reached the patients.

None of these conditions resulted from neglect or a serious shortage of funds but simply through ignorance, poor planning and bad management.

Straightaway, the new Superintendent increased the number of domestic staff.

She ordered a hot water system to be installed. And in a passage outside the kitchens, a dumb-waiter type of lift was built on which food could be quickly hoisted to the upper floors.

At every bed, patients were to be provided with hand-bells to summon attention.

She sent to Embley Park for masses of old curtains she'd seen stored away in the attics. From these she had new curtains, chair and bed covers made in order to create a more homely atmosphere.

Engaging nursing staff was her biggest problem. Nurses were easy enough to attract but few were of the right calibre. They were all interviewed personally by Florence but only a small proportion of applicants was taken on.

Right from the start she intended introducing

the new nursing methods she'd learned in Germany as well as pioneering some ideas of her own.

Originally only Church of England "gentlewomen" were supposed to be admitted but Florence was adamant the Institute be open to women of all faiths.

When everything was ready and the first patients arrived, she turned her mind to finance and insisted that all supplies – medical and domestic – be bought in bulk at wholesale prices.

After the Institute was firmly established she made further savings by advocating home sewing, home cooking, the growing and preserving of fruit and vegetables, together with making their own wines, meat spreads and jam.

The committee hadn't expected any of this. Their idea of a Superintendent was someone to carry out their orders and they thought she was a bit of a dictator. But they changed their minds when, within a few months, she managed to save them £150 – the equivalent of thousands of pounds today.

Florence was a "working" Superintendent, doing much of the actual nursing herself rather than delegating it to others. The patients adored her.

A lot of them were elderly and suffered from the cold – a discomfort Florence was personally familiar with – so it wasn't unusual to see her going from bed to bed, gently massaging numbed hands and feet back to living warmth.

Besides all this work and responsibility, she was still getting up at dawn studying statistics and hospital administration.

Some months after she'd moved into Harley Street, cholera – a highly infectious disease with vomiting, diarrhoea and agonising cramps – broke out in Soho, a notorious area of London's low life.

Hearing that the Middlesex General Hospital's resources were stretched to full capacity, she went to help and found herself nursing the worst kind of people her family had ever imagined: dirty, drunken, criminal, immoral.

Some were so dirty, lice could be seen crawling through their clothes and hair and on their skin. But Florence calmly stripped off their filthy garments and proceeded to apply turpentine poultices to their evil-smelling bodies.

She worked day and night, often going forty-eight hours without sleep. Many patients died in her arms. Cholera is so virulent that in the days before antibiotics the patient usually died within five hours of becoming ill.

The epidemic lasted three months, by which time Florence was ill herself from exhaustion. Her family were at Lea Hurst, always her favourite home, so she wrote to Elizabeth Gaskell asking if she would like to go there for a few days. With Elizabeth as companion, Fanny and Parthe wouldn't get the chance to nag and criticize her and she would get a well earned rest.

A week later she was back at the Institute working as hard as ever.

A few months later, with all the improvements completed, nurses well trained in their duties, organization and administration running smoothly, she felt fulfilled. But with the challenge gone she also began to feel stifled.

She started referring to the place as "a little molehill" and hinted that what bit of responsibility she was left with had diminished to boring routine work.

Although she'd achieved a lot for the Institute for the Care of Sick Gentlewomen, it seemed so little to her. Could that be her life's work completed? she wondered. Was that the mission God had called her to? Surely it wasn't all He expected of her.

At age thirty-four there could be many years left of her life, but they loomed ahead and appeared almost as tedious as those spent within the confines of her family.

Detecting the familiar signs of restlessness in their friend, Sidney and Liz Herbert told her that King's College Hospital, also in London, was going to be rebuilt. As she was now a well-known authority on nursing and hospital administration it was likely she would be its new Superintendent.

But even as they spoke Florence was musing over something that had been fermenting in her mind ever since she went to Kaiserworth.

With her annual £500 allowance she could rent a suitable building as a sort of school and start a campaign to attract farmers' daughters and other respectable country girls into learning nursing. She believed it would offer them an independent lifestyle rather than the loveless marriages they often drifted into for security.

With this in mind and what the Herberts had just told her, ideas about her future were in a whirl and it didn't seem so bleak after all.

Ironically, events were taking place in the outside world that would prove to be the very beginning of Florence's true vocation.

For over a year, Tsar Nicholas I of Russia had been claiming it was his responsibility to protect all Christians in any lands under Turkish rule. These were vast territories including, among others, Albania, Syria, Bulgaria, Muldavia (now Romania), Egypt, Cyprus, Macedonia, parts of Iraq, Libya, Tunisia, Yemen, Lebanon and Palestine.

Sultan Abdulmecid I dismissed this claim and gave his word that all Christians were perfectly safe under his rule and that the Tsar was interfering. In July 1853, the Tsar countered this accusation by sending his troops into Muldavia, a move which forced the Sultan to declare war on Russia.

All the while France and Britain were carefully monitoring the situation. They suspected Russia was intent on extending her territory right into the Ottoman Empire and using the protection of Christians as an excuse. A few weeks later, when a squadron of Turkish ships was destroyed in the Black Sea, both Britain and France entered into the conflict, demanding that the Tsar withdraw from Muldavia. Their demand was ignored so in March, 1854, they too declared war on Russia.

Since defeating Napoleon Bonaparte at Waterloo forty years earlier, Britain had been at peace. Now, with the fickleness of nations and politics, her army was fighting alongside the French.

Like most wars, this one wasn't taken seriously at first with everybody believing the "skirmish" would be over in weeks. But unlike most other wars, from the very beginning, this one was a fiasco of incompetence, wrong orders, mistaken orders, farcical organization, pomposity and general bungling.

In June, under the command of ageing Lord Fitzroy Raglan, 30,000 British troops landed on the western shore of the Black Sea at Varna, about 150 miles north of Constantinople, now Istanbul. They were joined by 30,000 French troops and there they stayed for the next three months waiting to be called into action.

The summer heat was intolerable yet uniforms were of standard issue and their living conditions quite insanitary. Not surprisingly, within weeks cholera broke out.

In September, just when the sickness was at its worst, orders came to prepare for battle. They were heading for Kalamita in the Crimea, 300 miles from Varna across the Black Sea.

Crammed on board scarcely seaworthy vessels, for lack of space the ailing army was forced to leave behind all medical supplies and most of its rations of salt pork and hard biscuits. Soldiers weren't allowed to take their kitbags containing personal belongings and bedrolls. Not even food for the pack-horses was loaded.

A hilly terrain in southern Russia, the Crimea is a peninsula jutting out into the Black Sea and connected to the mainland by such a narrow strip of land as to be almost an island in itself.

The voyage took days during which many died and their bodies were flung over the side.

They landed on 14th September with plans to advance on and lay siege to the big naval port of Sebastopol on the west coast of the peninsula. In the next four days dozens more died and 1,000 men were so sick they had to be put back on the ships.

The rest could hardly walk let alone fight, but

on 20th September, with sick men falling in their tracks, the attack commenced. In bright scarlet and gold-braided uniforms the vastly reduced numbers set off for the River Alma to the accompaniment of military bands. By some miracle, the Battle of the River Alma, north of Sebastopol on the west coast of the peninsula, was won by the allies – but with heavy casualties.

William Howard Russell was the London *Times* war correspondent who had journeyed with the troops. To get first-hand knowledge of conditions and how the fighting was proceeding, he lived alongside them in their inadequate tents which often lay in a foot of water.

Telegraph was now the modern method of communication. This ensured that his reports appeared back in Britain within a day rather than weeks or months as in the past. On reading his first account on 9th October the people were horrified.

Russell reported that, as well as being short on supplies, British troops were being "nursed" by old army pensioners while France had sent fifty Sisters of Charity to care for her soldiers. Weren't there any women in Britain able to come out and help? he demanded to know.

A second report appeared on 12th October and another the following day.

The British public had never before been given

graphic accounts of war. They were accustomed to rejoicing in the glory of military music and magnificent cavalry, the gallantry of men in colourful uniforms marching off to fight hundreds or thousands of miles from their homeland. But in this war they were spared nothing.

The Times contained details about the disgusting conditions the army was living in: food shortage, poor shelter, filth, torrential rain and mud which would be followed shortly by snow and freezing ice. Clothing that had been too heavy for the summer months was going to be inadequate for the severe Russian winter.

Neither medical nor any other supplies were being distributed as administration lay in chaos. Power of authority took precedence over soldiers' physical needs.

Adding to all this humiliation they'd had to rely on the French helping to carry both British and Russian war-wounded from the battlefields in their ambulances – covered carts drawn by horses, sometimes by men.

The newspaper report also related gruesome aspects of death, amputations and other kinds of woundings. And there was sickness: cholera, typhus (a fever caused through body lice) and gangrene (rotting flesh). All were brought on mostly through negligence.

For the first time, the British public felt personally involved in the struggle. Those terrible conditions they read about prevailed *now*, not many weeks in the past. There was public outrage that young men, fighting to protect the rights of Christians, should be so mistreated by their own people.

Very old ladies, barely able to care for themselves, came forward eager to go and tend boys young enough to be their own grandsons.

John Delane, *The Times* editor, organized a War Fund.

Appeals were made all over Britain for clothing, food and medical supplies along with medical personnel to be sent out immediately.

6.

BALAKLAVA

At the beginning Florence hadn't considered offering to help in the Crimea because, like everybody else, she hadn't expected the conflict to last. And anyway, female nurses hadn't been allowed inside military field hospitals since 1832. It was too impractical to provide transport for moving them around the battlefields and accommodate them under canvas.

But, she reasoned, if as the reports said there was a hospital building and an army barracks being used as a hospital at Scutari (now Uskudar) in Turkey, those rules would surely be changed and she was determined to go.

Her first task was to find a capable nurse as companion and when a Lady Forester heard about this she donated £200 to finance taking an extra *three* nurses.

In the new coalition government under the premiership of the Earl of Aberdeen, the Duke of Newcastle was Secretary of State *for* War while Sidney Herbert had become Secretary of State *at* War.

On 15th October, Florence wrote to Liz Herbert telling of her intentions. Did she think Sidney would support her and explain to the relevant authorities her age and moral reputation and how experienced a nurse she was?

By sheer coincidence, her letter crossed in the post with one from Sidney himself. He told her of all the incompetence he was encountering in Britain and assumed the same conditions prevailed in Turkey.

Every order he gave for supplies to be sent out had to pass through four official departments where they waited for days to be dealt with. Most got lost in transit and if an order managed to get through to the shippers, and if it was read, the supplies were packed up in crates and sacks, then left to wait on the quayside until some ship happened to be going in the right direction.

He ended by saying Florence was the only person he could trust to supervise and organize everything at the other end. Would she, please, go in the capacity of Superintendent?

Florence knew, with all the power and influence that lay in his grasp, she would get support from every source – not least from the British public. She immediately agreed, adding that she also wanted to take some nurses with her.

Within hours of receiving her reply, arrangements were under way. The Government approved and on 18th October appointed her with the grand title of Superintendent of the Female Nursing Establishment of the English General Hospitals in Turkey. She would come under the direct orders of Dr Menzies, Scutari's Chief Medical Officer, who would provide her with every facility and assist her to carry out her duties.

The Government funded the mission with £1,000 and donations from several individuals started coming in.

Charles and Selina Bracebridge, knowing that part of Europe well, were Florence's first volunteers. They helped to form an organizing committee consisting of themselves, Lady Stratford Canning, wife of the British Ambassador in Constantinople, and Miss Mary Stanley, the Dean of Westminster's sister.

Recruiting nurses was a different matter. Florence remembered the difficulty in getting suitable ones for the Institute in Harley Street.

Her nurses would get a uniform, free food and bed and be paid one shilling a day.

They wouldn't be permitted outside the hospital unless accompanied by at least three other nurses, and any found behaving in an immoral manner would be put on the first ship and sent home.

They must not wear jewellery, coloured ribbons or any other manner of adornment.

They would be allowed to drink only one and a half pints of ale or stout each day and one glass of brandy at night.

The Herberts offered the loan of their palatial Belgrave Square home in London for holding interviews. Seventy women applied out of whom only fourteen were accepted, and those more from desperation than suitability.

Florence approached the religious orders next and enrolled eight Sellonite Sisters, members of a Protestant order founded by a deeply religious Miss Sellon from Devonport in Kent. They were precisely the sort of women she wanted because they'd nursed cholera victims during the Soho epidemic. Also, part of their doctrine was never to shrink from dirt nor turn away from unpleasant sights – blood or mutilations, for example. And they must willingly accept every manner of hard labour at all times.

Five Roman Catholic nuns came from a convent in Bermondsey. From another Roman Catholic order came five who had only experienced nursing children in an orphanage.

There were Church of England sisters and some Elizabeth Fry nurses who had now changed their title from Sisters of Charity to the Institute of Nursing Sisters.

In all, the hand-picked team was made up of thirty-eight middle-aged nurses. Twenty-four of them were nuns with a mixture of Roman Catholic, Church of England and non-conformist.

None of them had experienced the horrors of war victims with their inevitable appalling injuries, but neither had Florence.

Having so many religious women in her party created another problem, for the government had stipulated that none of the nurses must try to impose her religion on any of her patients. And it was a well-known fact that some religious orders did just that. They believed their first duty was to save a man's soul and tend to his physical needs second.

Writing to Clarkey, Florence expressed her concern about this, adding that she wouldn't have such worries with the secular nurses. But Clarkey in reply joked that if they were like most nurses she knew, they would still have a deity to worship – Bacchus, the god of wine.

In view of the poor reputation nurses had, to lend respectability to their mission, uniforms – or livery as Florence called it – were provided. Hastily put together in a matter of days, they were ugly, ill-fitting and uncomfortable. They were grey tweed dresses with matching jackets and a short woollen cloak, with a white linen cap and a white scarf for round their shoulders bearing in red stitching the words Scutari Hospital. The nuns were more fortunate as they were permitted to wear their habits.

Florence was assured that everything at Scutari had been well prepared in advance, months earlier in fact. Doctors numbered one per every hundred patients. They would find plenty of medical and domestic supplies. Tons of lint had been despatched along with 15,000 pairs of sheets. Fresh meat, fruit and vegetables were leaving England's shores daily. Conditions were ideal.

However, in view of what Sidney Herbert had confided over how his supply orders were really handled, in the days leading up to their departure, Florence amassed bedding, socks, shirts, soap and towels together with as many medical supplies as she could get.

She planned to go on ahead of the group and her uncle, Sam Smith, aunt Mai's husband, was going with her as far as Marseilles.

Florence was extremely calm and composed in the face of the enormous task facing her – until the day before she left for Scutari when three letters arrived for her. The first she'd expected. It was an introduction to Dr Menzies at the military hospital.

The other two she wasn't prepared for. A letter from her mother gave Florence her blessing. At last, Fanny said, she realized the importance of her work. The change of heart was mainly because her daughter was growing famous.

The third was from Richard Monckton Milnes

who also gave his blessing. In it he jested that if she'd wanted to undertake such heavy responsibility she should have married him. From the tone of the letter it was obvious he still loved her and Flo must have felt the same way because she tucked it in her pocket and kept it with her always.

She couldn't decide what to do with Athena, the owl she'd tucked into her pocket all those months ago. But the problem was solved for her. That morning the little bird was found dead in its cage and only when she saw its pathetic little body did Florence betray all her pent-up emotions and anxieties and burst into tears.

With her uncle and a Mr MacDonald, who was in charge of *The Times* War Fund, she left England for France on 21st October and was seasick until the steamer landed at Boulogne. From there they travelled to Paris to await their companions.

Two days after Florence left, escorted by Charles and Selina Bracebridge, the rest of the Nightingale party, as it was known, set off from London by train for Folkestone in Kent and quite a crowd gathered to cheer them on their way.

When they met Florence in Paris, she astonished some of the nurses by purchasing a crate of eggs to ensure the Roman Catholics wouldn't have to eat meat as it was a Friday. They'd really expected her to be a harridan of a woman who would consider such observations humbug.

From Paris the entire party proceeded to Lyons from where they sailed down the Rhine to Valence, and from there by train to Marseilles.

Before starting on their final leg of the journey, they invested a large portion of the War Fund which had grown to £30,000. Florence bought some portable stoves to take with them and had everybody fitted out with warm, lined boots in readiness for combatting the winter. The secular nurses couldn't believe her kindness, saying no one had ever treated them so well before.

Then when they were ready to leave, news came through about the biggest blunder of the entire war – the ill-fated Battle of Balaklava.

Eight miles south-west of Sebastopol, defended by a ring of hills overlooking its little harbour, Balaklava had seemed ideally situated as a supply port for the allies. So secure in fact that Lord Cardigan, the Light Cavalry commander, had sailed his yacht into port and planned to live on it throughout the campaign, even bathing and dressing for dinner each night.

On 25th October, the Russians, hoping to breakthrough and relieve the great port of Sebastopol, attempted to attack the supply base. But they were driven back over a low ridge of hills by Sir Colin Campbell's 93rd Highlanders and the British Heavy Brigade under the command of Sir James Scarlett.

Mounted on his steed and looking down from a good vantage point on the Sebastopol heights, 66-year-old Lord Raglan saw that in their withdrawal the Russians had captured some heavy Turkish artillery. Seeing they were preparing to drag it away he sent his aide-de-camp down the valley ordering Lord Lucan, the cavalry commander, to send Major General Lord Cardigan's Light Cavalry in pursuit to "prevent them from taking the guns".

When Lord Lucan looked up at the hills, the only guns he could see were the Russians'. The captured artillery was concealed over a lower ridge on the Vorontson heights.

Knowing it would send them on a suicide mission Lucan thought he'd misunderstood the command and sent the aide back to clarify it. Raglan, of course, couldn't understand why he was being questioned and re-issued the order.

Gallantly the Light Calvalry, with the Heavy Brigade bringing up the rear, charged a mile and a half up the valley thinking they were expected to capture the Russian guns and rode straight into their heavy fire. The attack lasted a mere twenty-five minutes but of the 673 men who took part in the Charge of the Light Brigade, 478 were killed.

When news of the disaster was released, France's General Bosquet said, "It was magnificent but it is not war."

The British public was in uproar and demanded courts martial.

Alfred Lord Tennyson was moved to write two poems commemorating the tragedy, "The Charge of the Heavy Brigade" and the better known "The Charge of the Light Brigade".

Two days later, on 27th October, after saying farewell to her uncle, with a mixture of apprehension and stoicism Florence ushered her group on board the little vessel that was to take them the rest of their journey, lasting two weeks.

Vectis was a disgustingly filthy ship with cockroaches running everywhere. The weather was atrocious and water gushed down from the decks into their cabins which were inches deep in water. Every one of them was ill. No one ate for days and the crew seemed to forget they were on board so no one took them drinks.

On 29th October a gale blew up with towering waves threatening to capsize the little ship. They fell to their knees. Even non-believing nurses prayed for safe deliverance.

By the 31st, conditions were so treacherous that to keep from sinking, the crew had to jettison the guns. Terrible crashing sounds came from all around but by then, some were too ill to care and lay moaning on their cabin floors that were awash with ice-cold sea-water.

Late in the afternoon of 4th November, the winds died down and all movement of the ship suddenly stopped. Although it was raining hard, filled with terror, everyone staggered on deck to see what had happened. To their joy they were anchored in Constantinople harbour and were looking out at glittering minarets, brightly painted houses and beautiful gardens.

That evening, in groups of four, they were rowed across the narrow stretch of water to Scutari in *caiques*, beautifully carved gondolier-like boats in which passengers recline on huge cushions. For a few moments Florence thought wistfully of Venice and the Grand Tour but then they arrived at Scutari. It was just three weeks after Russell's first articles appeared in *The Times*.

As they approached land a terrible foreboding fell over the group as a great, ugly, yellow-walled building came into view. It was square with a tower at each corner and bore a strong resemblance to a medieval prison. It was the converted barracks "hospital".

A dead horse lying at the water's edge was being ravished by a snarling pack of starving dogs. There was no one to meet them at the jetty. A few native Turks, some soldiers and their wives stood watching and all looked as weary and dishevelled as the newcomers.

Thoroughly worn out, the little band trudged
up the hill to the hospital.

7.

SCUTARI

On entering the hospital and seeing the conditions, exhausted as they were, straightaway the women removed their cloaks and bonnets and rolled up their sleeves ready for work.

But although they were received courteously, it was made quite clear they weren't wanted.

The new arrivals were housed in six tiny rat- and flea-infested rooms in a turret high up on a bleak gable. Windows were broken and there were neither curtains nor shutters. There was no furniture, not even beds, but some orderlies came in with some rough blankets to put on the floors. A few rusting bowls were scattered about to catch the rain coming in through the ceiling.

They were glad they'd brought soap and towels but then learned they had an allocation of only one pint of water each per day for drinking and washing in. They had no cooking facilities save the little stoves bought in Marseilles but there was no food anyway.

As for nursing, they were banned from setting foot in the "wards" – corridors of the building, really – but they were told they could make bandages out of a few old sheets if they wanted to be useful, just so long as they kept out of the way.

Lord Napier, a Secretary from the British Embassy at Constantinople, came later that day to welcome them and found Florence lying on a couch, utterly fatigued and barely able to greet him.

The hospital stood on a steep hill, four storeys high at the front but only a single storey high at the rear. It was originally meant to accommodate 1,700 men but since the Battle of Balaklava, had nearer 4,000.

Harassed doctors and ward orderlies – made up of old men and soldiers recovering from wounds – were too busy to be bothered with the "ladies". They would be more of a nuisance than assistance.

This Miss Nightingale, they concluded, had obviously inveigled her way to Scutari through knowing powerful and influential people from her own social circle. She probably believed nursing meant administering cool hands to feverish brows and giving sips of water to grateful, smiling patients.

What did women of her background know of war or nursing, and especially of nursing vulgar soldiers with appalling wounds? They would be fainting from shock and littering up the place.

Not wishing to antagonize doctors or army officers, Florence instructed her nurses to do absolutely nothing without first getting official approval. If on passing the end of a ward they heard a dying man begging for water, they must pass by.

The women rebelled against this but Florence was a strict disciplinarian. She knew it was the only way to gain the confidence of those in charge and eventually gain entrance into the wards. If they argued or defied the authorities in any way, they could all be sent home.

In the next few days it was so frustrating to spend time sorting out the bed linen, towels and bandages they'd brought with them while only a matter of yards away, men suffered and died.

Florence soon discovered it wasn't wounds that most died from but disease and complications aggravated by dirt, malnutrition and general neglect. That very week, because necessary landing documents hadn't been signed, an entire ship's cargo of vegetables had gone rotten and been thrown into the sea.

North-east of Sebastopol on 5th November, the day after the Nightingale party had arrived, the great Battle of Inkerman was fought in dense fog. In less than two weeks its hundreds of casualties started coming in.

Many soldiers had their uniforms ripped from them in the battle and were near naked. Sick or wounded, shivering and suffering from frost-bite, they'd been packed into all kinds of crude vessels. Lying on straw mattresses, sometimes on the open deck, they were brought 300 miles across the Black Sea on which they were pitched and tossed about, then into the Bosporus Sea to Constantinople from where they'd sailed across the narrow strait to Scutari.

On their arrival they faced the same climb up to the hospital as Florence and her group had two weeks earlier. These men were dreadfully wounded or sick, yet there were no ambulance wagons or even stretcher parties. Those who were able staggered up the muddy banking helping to carry men who couldn't move at all. Others had to crawl to the top as best they could.

Lots had died on the voyage and of those who hadn't, gangrene was rife and hundreds more were destined to die. Some were in shock and speechless but those fit to communicate informed the hospital that hundreds more were on their way.

It didn't seem possible but beds were jammed together even more tightly.

That week a storm at sea sent two merchant ships to the bottom with a loss of winter clothes and medical supplies, including ambulance wagons.

Doctors and orderlies worked day and night

until, in desperation, on 14th November they had to call on Florence for help. Her own army had been waiting silently in the shadows for just such a moment. Immediately the word was given, they moved into the wards – and the doctors realized their worst fears.

Florence's behaviour and that of her charges over the past days had been exemplary and had lulled them into believing she would defer to their every command.

Resorting to her previous experience at the Institute, Florence was determined to bring a semblance of order to the chaotic organization. During their voyage one nurse had asked "Miss Nightingale" not to let officialdom stand in the way of nursing when they arrived. Florence, having some idea of what to expect, replied that she felt the hardest work would be done at the washtubs. She was right.

The place was incredibly filthy and so damp that condensation flowed down the walls. It ran onto the floor where patients lay on wooden pallets, their straw mattresses damp, sometimes soaked with blood and urine.

Open sewers ran under the great ugly building. All the lavatories were blocked and open tubs had been placed in every ward into which all body waste was tipped. The tubs were never emptied and the stench from the sewers, lavatories and those tubs pervaded the entire hospital.

There were four miles (6km) of passages acting as hospital wards, each one hopelessly overcrowded. Blood, pus, vomit, urine and excrement caked the walls and floors where all sorts of vermin and insect life thrived. And there wasn't a single scrubbing-brush throughout the building.

Men were suffering terribly, not only from wounds and sickness but from the bitter cold weather because they were half naked having lost everything. In the kitbags they'd been told to dump before sailing for the Crimea were their clothes, knives, forks and spoons. Now they had nothing and although the military store was full of everything they needed, no one had authority to give it out.

There was starvation too. Some moaned in their misery while others had passed beyond the awareness of it. They were both numb and dumb from shock, cold, hunger, sickness and pain. And the only ease for their suffering was the fact their voyage was over. They weren't being tossed about and they were under shelter.

Florence ordered that all the men be washed, their wounds cleaned and dressed, then they were to be put in clean beds. That night they slept. But as days went by, every patient who had been brought in that day died. She prayed to God, asking, was this her role, to ease their passing rather than help to heal them?

The first priority after that dreadful day of endless admissions was to see that all the lavatories were unblocked. Regarding the big tubs in the wards, she got the strongest ward orderlies to make improvised yokes by threading poles through the handles then carry them out slung between them on their shoulders.

Her next objective was to see that all foul bedding be washed. Until then only seven shirts had been washed and they were simply dipped into cold water then left to dry. They returned with the seams still full of lice. Men refused to have their shirts laundered, preferring to keep their own vermin than wear someone else's.

With some of the £30,000 from *The Times* War Fund she'd already rented a nearby building for use as a laundry and ordered copper boilers to be installed. When this was done she employed soldiers' wives to do the laundry.

Mr MacDonald went to Constantinople and bought bathtubs, bedpans, cutlery, socks, nightshirts, razors, scissors and all sorts of things – together with yards of sackcloth and two hundred scrubbing brushes for cleaning floors and walls.

Every surface was to be washed. But before the floors could be scrubbed, it took many wheel-barrow loads to remove the filth lying around. Hands ended up red raw both from the hard work and the liberal quantities of harsh soda and lye put in the water to counter the dirt – there were no detergents then.

Germs hadn't been discovered at that time either, so no one could understand Florence's preoccupation with cleanliness.

She ordered carpenters to make wooden frames and her women sewed some old sheets together then tacked them to the frames to make screens for surrounding the beds. This enabled the men to retain a degree of dignity.

Until then, they had no privacy while performing bodily functions or having painful wounds dressed. Even worse, all surgery was performed in the open ward. Everybody witnessed the horror of amputations and saw discarded limbs lying on the floor awaiting removal – all this while waiting for their own operations.

Fortunately, despite the shortages of everything else, chloroform was in plentiful supply so most patients were spared the agony that once accompanied the most minor surgery.

There was one exception to this. One of the doctors was opposed to using anaesthetics, claiming that he preferred to hear a man bawl lustily under the knife as it indicated he was still alive.

Sadly, Florence had no power to interfere. Strapped to the table, pleading eyes gazing up into hers, the terrified patient waited for his ordeal to begin. Florence could have run and hidden away until it was all over but she disciplined herself to stand beside him, hands folded in front of her, ready to face the ordeal with him. She exuded an air of serenity while her inside churned and she was in mental torment.

Men coming in from the battlefields were starving and told of how they'd eaten roots clawed from out of the frozen ground with their bare hands. They wouldn't fare much better at the hospital.

There was an enormous kitchen in the cellar but to feed those thousands of men there were only twelve ovens. And the food was quite unsuitable for anyone let alone invalids. Men who should have been on liquid diets were given the most revolting solids.

There were no cooks but orderlies hacked lumps of meat from animal carcasses and flung them into huge cauldrons on the stoves. This "meat" included bone, fat, gristle, eyes, ears and the rest. The pieces were thrown in at various times in the day but were all taken out at the same time. The meat put in first was so overcooked it dissolved from the bones. In that case it was the bones the patient got. The last pieces to be put in were taken out when only barely warm let alone cooked and this raw meat was also distributed.

But all food was given out only after two doctors had signed for it. When one signature was obtained, the other doctor was often nowhere to be found. Most patients couldn't eat anyway. They should have been on milk or arrowroot drinks for bowel disorders which most suffered from – today they would be on drips. Others had lost all their teeth and had gum disease.

When the Ambassador's wife called at the hospital to ask a nurse how the patients were, she was told, "As well as dying, starving men can be."

When Lady Stratford demanded to know what she meant by "starving" she was invited to tour the hospital and was so distressed she never returned. But from then on she sent regular supplies of nourishing calves foot jelly.

Scurvy was breaking out too because barrels of lime juice had been lying unopened for two months in the storeroom. This prompted Florence and Mr MacDonald to go out into the forbidding market-place in Scutari village and buy fresh fruit and vegetables.

Coffee was made from raw beans as 3,000lbs of tea hadn't been unpacked.

Pack-horses were literally starving to death yet there was as much fodder as they needed in the area – but no one had been authorized to buy it. At times, of the two – Russia and military authority – it seemed Russia was the lesser enemy.

Everything was done "by the book" causing some quite ludicrous situations.

Doctors had divided the building up into individual "regimental hospitals" and attended only to men from that regiment. If only fifty patients were in their section, they tended to them while another doctor could be coping with hundreds from his regiment.

Dr Menzies, Florence's immediate superior, soon realized how futile this arrangement was. But as throughout the whole of the campaign, bureaucracy reigned over common sense. Rather than redistribute patients or doctors himself, he'd sent to London to ask what the ruling was on such a move. Weeks later, after officials had scoured files, word came back that there were no rules covering such an event. But as everybody had to follow regulations, if none existed then nothing could be done, so the ridiculous situation stayed.

One, Dr McGreggor, scorned the ridiculous rules imposed on him and when a precious consignment of bed-linen, bedpans and other essentials arrived, he had them distributed straightaway to all the wards. But because they hadn't been processed with the appropriate documentation they were all re-collected and confiscated.

When it was found out that another doctor had issued milky gruel and wine to his patients, he was despatched to the Crimea the next day.

The portable stoves Florence bought at Marseilles had been installed at intervals throughout the wards so that nourishing hot drinks could be made all day long. But when the Deputy Inspector General of Medical Services saw them he had them removed as cooking in the wards was banned. Army orders must be obeyed at all times even though dying men begged for a warm drink. And this in wards that had seen so much squalor and deprivation only days earlier.

It was actually stated that patients' care came secondary to obeying regulations.

When 27,000 shirts and vests were shipped in from Britain, they couldn't be distributed until they'd been officially released by the Board of Survey. But the Board wouldn't be meeting for another three weeks so Florence bought 15,000 shirts out of her own pocket and gave them out instead. As they were her own personal property, the rules didn't apply.

There were times when she felt less like a nurse than a general dealer running a store. Always she was giving out bed-linen, clothes, food, cutlery to eat it with, even furniture, operating-tables, bedpans and commodes.

She rarely ate from morning till night. Sometimes she grabbed a bite to eat in the morning while walking about.

Although the women were proving themselves invaluable, far from showing gratitude, army doctors and officials were furious at all the interference. They hindered progress at every step and treated the nuns and nurses abominably, reducing some to tears.

To ensure none of her women could be accused of immoral behaviour Florence banned them from entering wards after eight o'clock at night.

In their letters home, nurses and nuns described the wonderful work Miss Nightingale was doing in such awful conditions. The family of one Protestant sister, Elizabeth, had her letter published in *The Times* to verify what William Russell had said.

When the military authorities in Scutari learned of this they demanded that sister Elizabeth should be questioned, claiming she'd lied. At her enquiry it was found that in her letter she'd mistakenly given the wrong number of dead. For that she was condemned as dishonest and untrustworthy and ordered home on the next ship.

Florence was very upset at losing one of her best nurses but she was amused when another asked to go home at the same time.

This nurse had come to Scutari prepared to

face anything and didn't mind the cold or the hard work but she felt she couldn't stay as her uniform hat didn't suit her.

After this, four of the nuns quarrelled with Florence over her harsh rules and asked to be sent back to England. All the other nurses saw her as a hard taskmaster too but they respected her.

The authorities thought she was a monster but the patients thought she was a saint.

She is often portrayed as solemn and humourless but on the contrary, Miss Nightingale was a lot of fun. In the midst of horror and squalor she liked nothing more than to make her colleagues and patients laugh.

Every night, her lantern gently swaying from side to side, she walked alone through all four miles of corridors, stopping from time to time to comfort a patient suffering great pain. When men saw the glimmer of her lamp and heard the soft rustle of her skirts approaching from the darkened corridors they felt an angel was in their midst. And at each makeshift bed, men kissed her shadow when it fell across them.

Although Flo never asked them to refrain from coarse language, never a swear word was heard in her presence, such was the love and respect these rough men felt for the Lady with the Lamp.

Such were her virtues that Richard Monckton

was told in a letter, "If the roof of the Scutari hospital opened and she was taken up, no one would be surprised."

She read and wrote letters for soldiers unable to do it for themselves. She also sat up late into the night writing letters of condolence to bereaved families, telling them their son, father, husband or brother had died in her arms.

Florence had a strict rule that no man must die alone. If he were unconscious, Selina would sit beside his bed until the last breath had left his body. But if he were conscious it was Florence herself who sat beside him, holding his hand, stroking his brow and talking soothingly right through to the end.

Some of the *men* were only sixteen. A man of thirty was considered "an old soldier".

A Scottish, golden, curly-haired bugle boy named Grant was no more than a child and kept asking for his mother. After the horrendous voyage across the Black Sea in pain he knew he was dying and thought he'd reached heaven when he was washed and laid in his bed by the tender women.

When nearing death, every man asked for his mother. And having softer hands than the rough orderlies, nurses hoped they died thinking she was with them.

8

THE LADY WITH THE LAMP

Queen Victoria followed events of the war closely and in a letter to her Secretary of State at War she asked Sidney Herbert to convey her gratitude to Flo and her ladies and ask them to pass on a message: "To the poor noble wounded and sick men that no one takes a warmer interest or feels more for their sufferings or admires their courage and heroism more than does their Queen. Day and night she thinks of her beloved troops. So does the Prince."

When Florence read out that part of the letter in each ward, the men were all touched and some were in tears.

Also in the letter, Queen Victoria asked if there was anything at all she could do. Florence didn't hesitate in asking if she could use her influence to get the rules on soldiers' pay changed. Wounded men lost 4d (2½p) a day, but a sick soldier had his pay reduced by 9d (4½p) per day, yet the sickness was as much the result of being at war as were the wounds.

Queen Victoria not only acted on this immediately, she also sent a shipload of goods for the men.

These consisted of water-beds, clothes, pipes and tobacco; writing paper and envelopes; sweets, biscuits, soap, wine and groceries; books and games.

Selina Bracebridge took charge of this Free Gift Store and distributed the commodities wherever and whenever they were needed. By this time, the British public were also donating gifts by the crate-load which were all added to the store.

William Russell, *The Times* war correspondent, was still in Turkey but was now sending home reports of a different sort.

But there were still some in authority who adamantly denied the truth of what he'd first reported. Like telegraphy, photography was another recent invention. So to prove Russell's lies they'd sent a photographer out.

Roger Fenton was never admitted entrance to the hospital at Scutari so he never had the chance either to prove Russell's reports false or to verify them. Instead, the military authorities dispatched him to the Crimea. He took 360 photographs during the campaign but none ever appeared in the newspapers. Most of his work was carried out in the battle zones. His "dark-room", a horse drawn, covered cart, stood stark on the bare landscape and could be seen for miles by friend and foe alike. Several times it was fired on but was always just out of range.

Only days before Florence arrived, Chaplain Osborne had reached Scutari intending to give spiritual comfort to the wounded and dying but he ended up aiding surgeons with amputations. He wrote to his close friend, Sidney Herbert, extolling the virtues of Miss Nightingale and her nurses and adding, "We could do with twice as many of their kind."

Although Florence knew Mary Stanley was continuing to enrol women, she'd made Sidney promise not to send any more out until she requested them. Now he wasn't sure. He was overworked and under stress. There were forty-four all eager to go so he gave permission.

Mary Stanley was going with them and her party was made up of fifteen Roman Catholic Sisters of Mercy, twenty so-called nurses and nine "ladies". They were an ill-chosen bunch with the "ladies" refusing to associate with the nuns because they were Roman Catholic, nor would they mix with the nurses who were, admittedly, drunk and foul-mouthed. All through the voyage there were quarrels and Mary Stanley had no idea how to discipline them.

They got to Scutari on 17th December, 1854, just six weeks after Florence who was by then getting everything nicely under control. Charles Bracebridge went with her to meet them at the jetty to tell them they couldn't stay. Some were drunk and so fat they'd nearly sunk the *caiques* on the way over from Constantinople.

Florence was very angry. She had been biding her time, gaining the trust of doctors and other officials with her well-behaved nurses. But these women didn't know her and wouldn't understand she was in a position to tell them what to do. On the other hand, Mary Stanley would expect them to do everything her way and she had no nursing experience whatever. Consequently they would be as useless as everybody had predicted her own group would be.

Giving them £15, she sent them to the Ambassador's home at Therapia about twenty miles away until she'd decided what to do with them. Mary returned a week later having run out of money. Florence lent her £100 and promised her a further £300 later.

They'd come out totally unprepared for the hardships ahead. Some time later the Stanley party was delegated to work at various hospitals. Some went to hospitals in the Crimea. Some were offered work in a naval hospital that was well managed because the navy wasn't very involved in the campaign and had fewer patients. Others went to a new 750-bed hospital at Kulilee, fifteen miles away. Florence learned later that conditions there were even worse than at Scutari.

Reports on their progress reached Florence's ears and were all she'd expected, especially regarding the "ladies".

They were so like her mother and Parthe doing their "ladies work". Dressed in finery all day long, they flitted about looking busy while actually doing nothing and squabbling the whole time. Most of the others were always drunk.

She was furious when she heard Mary had appealed to the British Ambassador for special food for herself as she found what was on offer in the kitchen at the hospital she'd been delegated to was unappetising. Yet the men in her care were starving. Mary Stanley couldn't stand the work or the weather so after a few weeks she was eager to leave.

Florence wrote to Liz Herbert asking to ensure that no more "ladies" came out to Turkey unless they were willing to get down to real work. There must be no drunkards and certainly no "fat old dames" as there was no room for them. But if Liz could personally select some good, responsible women, it wasn't a bad idea to have extra help.

Other than her own nurses, the only help came from orderlies who were a mixed bag of compassion, indifference and cold-hearted cruelty.

One patient, in gratitude for some small service, offered one of them 2s 6d (12½p), whereupon the orderly, seeing the glint of a sovereign in the man's pouch, struck him a blow on the head, killing him outright, then absconded with the pouch.

Some were caught one day playing leap-frog over the feet of dead and dying men. When reprimanded they claimed they were entitled to some fun and had to keep fit.

Surprisingly, some of the meekest, most grateful patients, on recovering and becoming orderlies themselves, turned out to be every bit as unkind.

In stark contrast there were others such as one old army pensioner who broke down crying, calling himself "a silly old fool" for not being able to do more. Yet he was doing everything possible to comfort the men in his care.

At Inkerman the Russians had lost 11,000 men and as the winter was getting its grip they gave up trying to relieve the seige on Sebastopol until the spring.

Not until winter was nearly over did warm clothing begin to arrive for the British troops.

At Balaklava, Russian soldiers had been seen wearing knitted helmets that covered the ears and neck with an opening for the face. These were described in letters home and soon, mothers, wives and sisters were knitting them and sending them out to the troops.

James Brudenell, the 7th Earl of Cardigan, commander of the Light Cavalry, always wore a knitted jacket which buttoned right down the front. When soldiers wrote home, they mentioned this sensible garment which they'd named "the cardigan" and they too were knitted and sent out.

Lord Raglan, the campaign commander, also unwittingly created a style. He had lost an arm at the Battle of Waterloo during the Napoleonic wars and found the thick shoulder seams in his army great coat were uncomfortable. To prevent chafing the still tender flesh, his tailor had made a coat with sleeves continuing right up to the neckband thus eliminating a shoulder seam altogether. On hearing about this in Britain, a lot of the knitted cardigans were made with "raglan sleeves".

As the New Year of 1855 came in, there were 40,000 soldiers in the Crimea of whom 25,500 were sick or wounded − and 12,000 of those were in the barracks hospital.

War wounds appeared to be lessening in their severity but sickness was rife and there were still more dying from disease than their injuries. In two weeks, four doctors died of typhus.

Bacteria had been discovered in the seventeenth century but it wasn't realized they caused disease. In 1847 a Hungarian doctor, Ignaz Semmelweis, had noticed that when he washed his hands in chlorine water between attending patients the death rate had fallen. But he didn't know why.

One progressive Scutari doctor was interested in this theory and had an orderly follow him from bed to bed with a bowl of water in which he washed his hands after seeing to each man. But as nobody had signed for a towel he wasn't allowed one so a nurse gave him a sheet of lint to dry his hands on. The same doctor also started using separate swabs for bathing each patient's wounds. Previously, one sponge had done for the whole ward.

None of this had any effect on the death rate though and all the other doctors scoffed at him.

It was ironic that men who had suffered amputation out on the battlefield, with little shelter and no anaesthetic, usually recovered, while those operated on in the hospital under chloroform deteriorated and died within days. This was because the men out in the field were fit at the time of being wounded. Those in hospital had endured the rigours of waiting days to start on a ten-day voyage to the hospital. By the time they reached it they were covered in fearful sores from being rolled about on deck. Some had all the skin taken off their back and this was more painful than their wounds. Their stamina was so low by then they hadn't the strength to survive surgery.

Men were dying day and night and the women became despondent. Hospitals should be places of healing, not just somewhere to die. They prayed that some would start to recover and make all their effort seem worthwhile. But it seemed all they could do was offer comfort until merciful death came along.

Florence was always being promised help from army officials and Embassy staff in Constantinople but none ever came.

Always having been easily depressed, there were times when she felt utterly alone. In a letter to Sidney Herbert she said that apart from him, the Bracebridges and herself, no one seemed to care.

He quickly replied that she should beware of putting such thoughts in writing lest they fall into the wrong hands. She still had opposition in high circles.

That winter 9,500 died in five months, 8,000 of them from cholera. At her wits end, Florence wrote to Sidney Herbert urging him to press for a government enquiry regarding the lack of supplies and the insanitary conditions at the hospital.

There was so much criticism of the government's handling of the war at that time that in

February 1855, the Prime Minister, the Earl of Aberdeen, felt obliged to resign and Lord Palmerston – Florence's old friend and neighbour, PAM – became premier.

The Duke of Newcastle also resigned as Secretary of State for War and Lord Panmure, later Earl Dalhousie, took the post.

Lord Panmure didn't know Florence but he'd heard so much from Sidney, he'd come to admire her. He was a diplomat who knew how to get his way without angering opponents and immediately ordered representatives to go to Scutari and conduct an enquiry. Whatever proposals they made for improvement were to be implemented at once under their personal supervision.

Dr John Sutherland led the enquiry and among his colleagues were a Health Inspector from Liverpool and a member of the Board of Poor Relief in Scotland.

When they arrived in April they found that the water supply was polluted from scores of rotting animal carcases lying in water all the way from its source right up to the hospital.

Twenty-five decomposing animal carcases were found lying in the hospital yard and around the outside walls.

Sewers under the building were swarming with rats.

Orders went out that the sewers were to be

flushed clean. Walls must be lime washed to eliminate further infestation from vermin and lice. No patient coming into the hospital was to be placed on an old mattress and soiled mattresses were to be burned.

A month after that massive clean-up operation, the death rate dropped from 42 per cent to 2 per cent but not before a further 2,000 men had died.

The winter lull in the fighting was nearing its end. As the snows began to melt and everywhere was covered in bitterly cold, sometimes knee-high, slush, the onslaught started again from both sides.

Deaths from disease had diminished but casualties were pouring in and the death rate soared above all previous numbers.

Corpses were always buried in their shirts and shrouded in blankets until the hospital started running short of them. Then orders were given that bodies could no longer be interred in blankets and must be stripped of all garments which were to be handed over to other patients.

When this got known in Britain, there was such an outcry at men being buried naked "like dogs", that fresh orders went out immediately for them to be wrapped in sacks.

Day after day, nurses stood at the windows watching burial parties trudging along to a makeshift cemetery on the hillside. The bearers were ward orderlies. There were no mourners, no coffins. From time to time the bearers would stop for a rest and lay their burden on the ground while they smoked a pipe, chatting and laughing before resuming their journey.

The dead were buried in huge square holes which, when nearly full, were shovelled over with a thin layer of earth then trampled down.

How that upset the watchers, knowing the heartache of families at home had they been aware of the callous indifference at their loved ones' passing.

In a small, quiet room, Florence and the Brace-bridges read prayers every morning with the nurses. The Roman Catholics had mass and walking wounded were able to attend either service. But while men who were confined to their beds were begging for prayers, chaplains weren't permitted to hold services in the wards "for fear of offending patients of varying faiths".

One Colonel, recovering from his wounds, found out that, being a soldier, the rule didn't apply to him so he took it on himself to go from ward to ward saying prayers.

Miss Tebbit, a young nurse of the Unitarian faith, discovered her own cousin was a patient in one of the wards. When she went to see him he asked if he could borrow a book of hers called *Christian Year*. When he'd finished reading it he placed it beside his bed where it was picked up by a chaplain who asked if he could borrow it.

Some days later when Miss Tebbit asked for it, she was told she'd broken the rules on proselytising – trying to convert people into her faith – and that he'd sent the book to the War Office to let them see what sort of bigotry was being preached at Scutari.

Whoever received the complaint at the War Office wisely ignored it. Months later, being an excellent nurse, Miss Tebbit was made Superintendent at another hospital.

Under Florence's guidance, the barracks hospital was cleaner and food – now weak broth made from boiled bones – had improved a bit but it still wasn't satisfactory. Her children, as she called her patients, deserved better.

She wrote to the very exclusive Reform Club that boasted one of London's best chefs and asked if he would come out to Turkey and teach the orderlies how to cook for invalids.

Alexis Soyer, a dapper little man, not only agreed to go but took four other chefs with him. After having all the ovens serviced he set about instructing orderlies in the cooking of meals. These proved so appetising and nutritious that patients cheered him whenever he went into a ward.

Rather than being doomed to die, soldiers were now recovering and they wrote home telling their families about Florence. Troops who were fully recovered and able to return to Britain were relating all she had done in a very short space of time.

Now the mortality rate had dropped, the hospital was cleaned and the food improved, Florence turned her mind to other improvements.

A recreation room was set aside for reading and writing. For those who were illiterate she put in a request for two teachers to be sent out. She also begged for books, exercise books, writing paper, pens, ink, games, footballs, chess sets and short play-scripts for the men to perform in drama groups.

Stuffy elderly officials were enraged. These "fighting brutes", as they called the soldiers, weren't deserving of such refinements.

Florence's next project was to get men to send home a percentage of their pay. This above all her ideas was heartily jeered at by the military authorities. They claimed that all soldiers wanted was to spend their money in the Turkish villages on drink, tobacco, gambling and immoral women.

They were proved wrong when in the first month almost £11,000 was sent home to parents, wives and families.

Florence was adamant she would change the attitudes of the military authorities. Soldiers must no longer be thought of as mere "gun fodder" – a dispensable lower form of human life. They risked life and limb in protecting their fellow human beings – the very society that often disapproved of them – and in future they must be given their due respect.

With everything nicely under control, she remembered hearing a wounded soldier describe Scutari as Paradise compared to Balaklava. Now it was time to go out to the Crimea and see the conditions for herself.

9.

THE CRIMEA

In the company of Charles Bracebridge, four nurses and Alexis Soyer, the London chef, Florence left for Balaklava.

They sailed on the *Sir Robert Lowe*. Being worn out and not feeling well to start with, she was ill for the 300-mile voyage across the Black Sea, reaching Balaklava on 5th May 1855. It was exactly six months to the day from her arrival at Scutari.

Once back on land Florence soon rallied and eagerly made plans to visit Lord Raglan, the Cavalry Commander. Over the months they had built up a strong friendship through correspondence but they'd never met. With baggage loaded on mules and camels they set off over the rugged terrain.

Forsaking her ugly, drab uniform, Florence had chosen a dark blue riding-dress and fetching blue bonnet. Riding a graceful, golden mare she looked positively regal.

Unfortunately, when they arrived at Lord Raglan's camp he was away inspecting his troops in a far-out post. Undaunted, Florence rearranged her plans and made for the trenches.

High above Sebastopol, troops were dug in ready to make a final assault on the great naval port. It was spring and the horrors of the past winter were almost behind them. Florence thought how sad it was that as nature would soon be throwing up new shoots of life, these young men were preparing to fight and possibly to die.

The soldiers had only heard of the lady with the lamp and expected to see an elderly, dour woman. Instead they saw a beautiful young woman of thirty-five with luxuriant, gleaming chestnut hair. She was of average height with a slender, girlish figure. Her grey eyes sparkled. She had the softest, soothing voice and a warm smile for everyone. All the same, no one doubted the aura of determination and tenacity below the surface.

Bravely she climbed up to the look-out post and for a while sat on the barrel of a huge cannon gazing out over the Russian lines. An officer told her that ladies frequently went up there to see the view and the enemy had never fired a shot while they were present. On this occasion, even as he spoke, a shot was fired and went right over their heads. Florence didn't flinch at the deafening cannonade nor did she leave until she was ready.

Unknown to her, while she was surveying the land, soldiers had collected bunches of lilies and orchids growing wild around the trenches. Five bunches in all were offered to her and she was asked to choose whichever one she liked best. Without a moment's hesitation, and to their immense delight, she swept them all into her arms.

There were four hospitals on the Crimea with some of Mary Stanley's nurses and some other new arrivals working in each of them and these were next on her itinerary.

At the first one, Florence wasn't happy with either the nurses' work or their manner and lack of discipline, particularly that of one, the Reverend Mother Bridgeman.

But when Florence reproached them she was told that her title was Superintendent of the Female Nursing Establishment of the Military Hospital of the Army in Turkey. As this was Russia, she had no authority over Crimean hospitals.

They also said they'd heard that at Scutari she took good care of herself while her nurses were left to starve.

Lord Raglan was furious when he heard this and wrote to the officials at the hospital in her defence. He reminded them she not only had his support but also that of the Prime Minister, Lord Palmerston, the Secretary of State for War and Queen Victoria herself.

At this her critics acquiesced and permitted her to make a full inspection of all four hospitals.

Wherever she went people were amazed at her appearance, yet she didn't even look her best. Like the soldiers at the front, they had expected a middle-aged amazon of a woman, stern, unfriendly, bossing everybody about and more concerned with the hospital than the patients in it.

When she walked among the men, stopping at each bed, enquiring of their injuries or illness, offering words of comfort and, for those well enough, leaving them chuckling over some remark, they understood how she'd inherited her unofficial title – the angel of Scutari.

She completed her inspection, giving ample praise where it was credited but not hesitating to point out what dissatisfied her.

Meanwhile, Alexis Soyer was conducting his own inspection and went about pinning invalid recipes on hospital kitchen walls.

Two weeks after reaching Balaklava, Florence came down with typhus – by then known as Crimean fever. It came on so suddenly, she had to be carried on a stretcher into the Castle hospital.

It was one Crimean hospital Florence had no criticism of. Under the supervision of Mrs Shaw-Stewart – the only one of Mary Stanley's party with any nursing experience – it was ideally managed.

For days, as the fever raged, she rambled incoherently.

The hardships of the last six months had sapped all her energy. In those days there was a belief that one's strength went into the hair and also that the brain needed cooling to offset delirium, so her beautiful long hair was cut very short. Still, doctors said it was too late, she couldn't survive.

Sometimes it was just possible to make out what she was saying in her delirium and it was always the same sort of thing. Quoting figures and statistics. Directing nurses in their work. Reeling off endless lists of supplies that were needed and lists of what had arrived. Numbers of dead. Numbers expected to die. Causes of death.

When news of her imminent death reached Scutari, even the most hardened men wept.

Late on the night of 24th May, Lord Raglan, himself an ailing man, rode miles from his camp to see her. When he saw how ill she was he slumped down in a chair but doctors assured him she was a little improved from that morning. For an hour he sat holding her hand but she kept drifting off into oblivion.

Incredibly, despite her frailty, once the fever broke, Florence made a quick recovery. Knowing fighting was likely to start at any time, she was eager to get back to Scutari to make preparations.

But everyone – doctors, the Bracebridges and Alexis the chef – insisted she must go home to England. Although she was feeling better, it would be months before she was fully recovered and she needed a long convalescence.

But Florence was determined to get back to Scutari.

Like Cardigan, Lord Ward also had his yacht anchored at Balaklava. And knowing how bad a sailor she was and how very ill she'd been, he came forward and placed the luxurious vessel at her disposal.

However, doctors and Charles told her she would be better sailing in a naval ship, *Jura*. Its size would make for stability, thus preventing sea-sickness. It was due to leave for England and would call in at Scutari for Florence to disembark.

She didn't know they'd worked a ploy. *Jura*'s captain had no intention of putting in at Scutari but was sailing directly to England. Once Florence was aboard, she would have to go home.

Whether she had some inkling of this will never be known but no sooner had she gone aboard when she began to complain of nausea and faintness. A large number of cavalry horses had just been disembarked and the holds where they'd been stabled were still waiting to be cleaned out. After what she had endured over the past months, the terrible stench rising from below wouldn't normally have bothered Florence but in her delicate state it was too much.

Of course, she had always been capable of inducing illness when it was expedient, so if she did suspect there was a ruse to get her back to England she would have employed the talent then. She was hastily transferred to Lord Ward's yacht.

As was expected, she was sea-sick throughout the twelve-day voyage. At Scutari she had to be carried ashore.

The welcoming party at the little jetty were shocked to see the change in her in such a short time: thin, pale, her hair all cut away, and so weak her voice could barely be heard.

She was taken to the Chaplain's house where she spent a period of six weeks' convalescence. At first she couldn't sit up or even lift a spoon. Doctors told her the fever had probably saved her life. She was at such a low ebb the enforced rest was what she needed.

The concern in Britain overwhelmed the Nightingale family who received thousands of letters all expressing their good wishes.

Sidney Herbert sent Florence a puppy and a

baby owl hoping a replacement for Athena would cheer her up.

When she was feeling much better, one of the soldiers' wives took her young baby each day and placed it in a sort of play-pen outside her window for her to watch it playing.

In the third week of that enforced rest Florence received news that put her recovery back for quite some time. On 28th June, Lord Raglan had died at Sebastopol after a very short illness. He had never recovered from the disastrous Charge of the Light Brigade knowing how many had pointed the finger of blame at him.

Florence was devastated that the sick, elderly man, when he thought she was dying, had ridden so far late at night to visit her little knowing he was so near death himself. And she thanked God that they had at least met on that one occasion.

In addition to losing a dear friend, she was further upset on learning that his replacement was General Simpson. He was known to share the same opinion as the Duke of Wellington who, at the Battle of Waterloo, was heard to say that soldiers were the scum of the earth. And, like the military authorities at Scutari, General Simpson was totally opposed to what he called "this new-fangled pampering of soldiers".

Another blow was to follow. Charles and Selina were feeling the strain. They too were getting old. The past months had taken a toll of their health and they felt they must get home to England. They tried all ways to persuade Florence to go with them but to no avail. They sailed on 28th July.

The following day Florence resumed work at the hospital where she was told that, as everything was running smoothly, she wasn't needed.

It was true the place was clean and men were recovering. But she could see that, in her absence, stupid bureaucracy and officialdom had taken a firm hold again. With the same fortitude she'd shown nine months earlier, Florence was determined to stay.

But all sorts of trouble lay in store for her.

Only a few of the nurses who had recently come out were living up to expectations. Some were getting hopelessly drunk and had to be sent home. Six of them married soldiers within days of getting there and never started work in the hospital.

The Free Gift Store that had been in Selina's charge until she left for home was now being very badly managed by a Miss Salisbury.

When Florence saw that a lot of stock was missing and wasn't recorded as being given out she started investigating and discovered it was all in Miss Salisbury's room. Every kind of item was crammed in cupboards, drawers and under her bed. But not only was it goods from the Free Gift Store but from the Government Issue stock as well. This was an even more serious offence.

Florence reported it immediately to the Military Commander, General Stork, an ardent admirer of hers. He had just replaced Lord Pault, one of the men who objected to all of Florence's reforms.

When General Stork threatened to have Miss Salisbury prosecuted, hysterical and prostrate on the floor, she begged for mercy and pleaded to be sent home. Neither the General nor Florence wanted it known that someone in their trust had been stealing the Queen's gifts and those of the British public so they let her go.

Once home, however, Miss Salisbury wrote to Mary Stanley telling her she'd been wrongly accused. It was Florence who wasn't allowing the gifts to be given out. She claimed she was neglecting patients and even intimated that she had caused the death of Miss Clough, one of the nurses.

The truth was that Miss Clough had been a thorough nuisance, awkward, always complaining, lying and often drunk. When she said she wasn't well and wanted to go home, although Florence believed it was a trick, she was pleased to let her go. But as soon as she got on board ship, Miss Clough took ill and died before it sailed. Her body was taken ashore where Florence arranged her funeral and wrote home to her family telling them what had happened.

Mary Stanley was jealous of Florence's achievements when her own endeavours had failed. Now she seized the opportunity for revenge.

She sent the letter to the War Office where there were still a number opposed to Florence's presence in Scutari.

WEN, Fanny and Parthe had been terribly anxious when Charles and Selina arrived back in England without Flo. So when they heard about all the trouble Mary Stanley was making they felt someone from the family ought to go out and give her support.

Aunt Mai Smith was the first to volunteer but uncle Sam and their children objected. She wasn't a young woman and she was needed at home.

Hilary Bonham-Carter seemed the next best choice as she and Flo were always fond of each other. Before she could be asked, though, aunt Mai had persuaded her family that if she went she would be back before the winter set in, so they agreed.

Mai Smith reached Scutari on 16th September and nearly collapsed when she saw her niece.

Pale and thin, her short hair beginning to curl round her face and ears, her grey eyes looking enormous in her pinched face, she looked like a little waif.

Like so many at home, Mai thought Flo's sole duties were nursing the men and giving out orders to subordinates. She had no idea how much she had to do.

She was writing letters, instructions, reports, compiling statistics and drafting out ideas for reforms that were badly needed in the British army. From getting up at 5 am, sometimes she worked right through until three or four o'clock the next morning. And still she made her nightly four-mile rounds of the wards.

On 8th September, 1855, the combined allies launched an all-out attack on Sebastopol and broke through the defences, causing the Russians to withdraw from the city. And although this victory heralded the end of the infamous Crimean War, it dragged on for a further six months.

In October, a month after the fall of Sebastopol, Florence declared herself fit enough to return to the Crimea and complete her hospital inspection.

At every hospital nurses, nuns, doctors and supervisors were quarrelling. All orders and instructions were altered or ignored. People were leaving their posts and usurping positions they'd no right to. Some even walked out of one hospital, into another and took over completely. When they'd disrupted that place they moved on again.

Nearly everybody concentrated on their own importance and fought over petty slights. No one seemed interested in the patients' welfare. It was absolute mayhem.

The biggest offender was the Reverend Mother Bridgeman – Mother Brickbats, Florence called her. She dismissed the fact that Florence was her superior and kept telling Florence what she must and must not do. She even ordered her to send some of her Scutari nurses over to the Crimea.

Although the weather was atrocious and she feared a bad voyage, Florence was glad when it was time to leave. Then as her ship made for the harbour mouth at Balaklava, freak winds stopped it getting through the narrow straight.

Because no one could be sure how long the ship would be stranded there it was decided that Miss Nightingale – already prostrate in her cabin with sea-sickness – would have to return to shore. As a small boat was brought alongside, a sailor picked her up in his burly arms and dropped her over the ship's rail into it. Tossed and flung about, she was taken back to Balaklava.

Days later, with the storm still raging, she took ill with sciatica – a painful, nerve-related inflammation in the hip and leg – and once more she ended up in the Castle hospital.

10.

STRIFE AND FAME – THEN PEACE

Florence was in hospital for only a few days, but in that time her world was tipped upside down.

Newspapers were sent out regularly to Turkey and the Crimea. They were about two weeks out of date by the time they arrived but everybody was eager to read the news from home.

While reading an old copy of *The Times*, but for the pain she was suffering, Florence would have leapt out of bed. There, glaring out from the page in front of her, was a report on a lecture that had been given by Charles Bracebridge, an account of his experiences in Scutari.

He'd made an outright attack on the military and medical authorities for their pomposity, incompetence, neglect and downright ill treatment of the troops.

But the virtues of Miss Florence Nightingale were extolled to a point where readers would infer she'd performed miracles.

The impression was that from her arrival at Scutari she had, single-handedly, healed thousands of men, tended thousands of dying men and, with *The Times* War Fund, rebuilt the hospital – and all in the space of about two days. Among many more accomplishments, she'd told ignorant doctors where they were going wrong and had innovated previously unimagined remedies.

Florence was so angry. In one fell swoop he'd undone all her good work. Her critics in the War Office, in the Scutari hospital and in the Crimea had been given fuel to fire their allegations of interference. Charles had also added credence to the lies and rumours her enemies seized on at every given opportunity. She felt like Jesus, betrayed by a trusted friend – albeit, in her case, a well meaning one.

Before she was well enough to leave Balaklava her predictions were in evidence. She was kept waiting for appointments. She was spoken to brusquely by officials while some people ignored her altogether and "Mother Brickbat" was elated.

Florence dreaded the reception waiting for her at Scutari from both military and medical authorities, especially now General Simpson was in command.

Still she had aunt Mai and General Stork's support as well as her nurses and some of the doctors.

By a strange quirk of fate, though, Charles's

account had an affect Florence hadn't anticipated. The British public had taken her to their
hearts. Her fame spread far and wide and within
days she'd become a national heroine.

Songs were composed in her honour and sung
everywhere from public houses to sombre choral
groups.

Music-hall artists reduced audiences to tears.

In every home where there was a piano or
organ, the sheet music was proudly propped up
on the music stand.

At church services, hymns were chosen in her
honour.

A book on her life was hastily written and
sold in the streets for one penny each. Within
days all copies were sold out.

Portraits of the Lady with the Lamp were
painted by people who had no idea what she
looked like.

Florence had suddenly become the most
popular name for baby girls.

Ships and a lifeboat were named after her.

Staffordshire figurines of "Miss Nightingale"
were produced.

And at Madame Tussaud's wax museum a
scene appeared depicting the Lady with the
Lamp bending over the bed of a stricken soldier.

The name of Florence Nightingale, the Lady
with the Lamp, was on everybody's lips.

But before news of this got circulated around

the Crimea, Florence had an urgent call to return
to Scutari where cholera had broken out. Once
more beds were rapidly filling up and deaths
occurring by the hour.

Over the past weeks, being so involved in
hospital management and general administration, nursing had been pushed aside. But
nurses and doctors were dying from the disease
so now Florence was back in the wards, doing
the job she loved most.

In the midst of the cholera outbreak, letters of
recognition from public figures and letters of
thanks from soldiers' families arrived daily.

Letters from WEN, Fanny and Parthe told her
they themselves were receiving dozens of similar letters. Total strangers were coming to the
door asking if they could see her writing desk.

In one delivery Florence received a package
bearing the royal cipher. Queen Victoria had
been so impressed by Charles's report, she'd
sent Florence a magnificent gift of a red enam-
elled oval brooch. Designed especially for her
by Prince Albert, it bore a crown and three stars
set with diamonds and was inscribed: VR.
Round the edge were the words: BLESSED ARE
THE MERCIFUL. At the base was one solitary
word: CRIMEA. On the reverse was engraved: To
Miss Florence Nightingale as a mark of esteem
and gratitude for her devotion towards the
Queen's brave soldiers from Victoria R 1855.

In England on 29th November, Sidney Herbert, Richard Monckton Milnes and the Dukes of Cambridge and Argyll formed a committee to find some way of showing the British people's gratitude to her. At a public meeting it was unanimously agreed that a Nightingale Fund should be formed to finance whatever project she chose.

Despite this acclaim, Florence's opponents openly declared that they agreed with all Miss Salisbury and Mary Stanley had said: that she interfered with the military authorities, behaved badly to doctors, ill-treated nurses and didn't care about the patients.

These accusations stemmed from petty jealousies in some quarters, from opposition to women having authority in others, while from others – mostly at the War Office – it was the belief that humane treatment for soldiers was misplaced. They were "animals", "brutes", "sots" and "scum".

To the consternation of Flo's critics, gleefully embracing every scurrilous word, the official report from the enquiry team that had been sent out to the barrack hospital was released. It was an impartial report and the facts confirmed the conditions reported in *The Times* by William Russell. They also refuted every complaint made against Florence.

Meanwhile, in Scutari the onset of winter had

eradicated the cholera and Florence was back at her writing-table.

Following the trouble from Miss Salisbury and Mary Stanley, she had been asked to send a detailed account of her side of the story. This alone involved writing a twenty-eight page foolscap document. She finished it early on Christmas morning.

Lord and Lady Stratford had invited Flo and Mai to lunch at the Embassy that day and Mai couldn't believe her ears when Flo agreed to go. When they arrived, dressed all in black, she was taken for a nun. She looked so ill, no one recognised her.

In the afternoon there was dancing and party games but Flo was too weak to join in. Still, her aunt was delighted to see her laughing so much at the antics that tears streamed down her cheeks.

Standing at her window in her spartan room that night, the roar of the ocean took her back to Lea Hurst and the rushing sound of the River Derwent. How far she had travelled since those days – and in so many ways. But, she told aunt Mai, she regretted none of it: the cold, hunger, illness or any of the misery she'd endured.

They faced a terrible winter of snow and gales. Badly fitted windows rattled and let in draughts, rain and snow. The little fire in Flo's room smoked so much it couldn't be lit. Seated back to back for warmth, Florence worked at her big table while aunt Mai worked at a smaller one. Always it was writing, writing and more writing.

Anxiously, Mai would implore her, "Flo, please to go to bed. Leave that for tomorrow."

But always, accompanied by a weak smile, she got the same response: "Tomorrow will bring its own work."

The only times she finished working before the early hours was when the ink froze solid in the ink-well.

In the following March, Austria threatened to enter the conflict, a move that brought about a speedy end to the war.

War's end, however, didn't mean everybody could simply pack up and go home the next day. Hospitals still had patients and men wounded in the last days of the war would shortly be arriving both at the Crimean hospitals and at Scutari after their 300-mile voyage across the Black Sea. And, of course, there were thousands of troops in camps scattered about the Scutari area and on the Crimea.

On 1st April, 1856, Florence arrived back at Balaklava to install ten Bermondsey nuns in the General Hospital and try to make peace with Mother Bridgeman now she'd brought over some extra nurses.

Mother "Brickbats", however, wouldn't have

anything to do with her, and after a confrontation, she and her nurses stormed out of the hospital.

Florence went to settle the nuns in the huts set aside as living-quarters that Mother Bridgeman and her party had just vacated, only to find them locked. The keys were held by Mr Fitzgerald, the store-keeper, and he'd gone into the town.

Although it was early spring, the Crimea was still in the grip of winter and on that day a blizzard was blowing. It was early in the afternoon when someone went in search of Fitzgerald. Florence was left standing outside the huts but the keys didn't arrive until the evening. By then she was numbed to the bone, tired and feeling ill.

The following day, however, she went with her nurses to the hospital to take up their duties and found it in a disgraceful state.

New kitchens that were supposed to have been in use by the previous November hadn't even begun to be built. One of Alexis Soyer's chefs had gone out weeks earlier but hadn't been allowed to work.

Patients were hungry and filthy dirty. Their beds crawled with vermin. A rat hovering in the rafters above a patient's bed was about to pounce when Florence spotted it and killed it with a stick.

Some patients had such appalling bed sores that their shirts and bedding was stuck to them. It took long, painful, harrowing hours to ease the clothing from them, cleanse their raw flesh and apply dressings. It took Florence and the ten nuns five full days to get first the patients then the building clean.

After that, she set out on another tour of inspection, visiting hospitals and military camps, often six and seven miles apart.

In one of the world's first ever war photographs Florence is seen standing on a windswept, snow-covered hill looking out to the Black Sea. Behind her stand rows of flapping grey tents housing the soldiers.

There were no roads in the Crimea, just rough tracks and she was on horseback for as long as ten hours a day. Sometimes it was nightfall before she got back. With only a lantern to guide her, she had to dismount and stumble through heavy snow.

Eventually she started riding in an open mulecart and was jolted and bruised but she didn't complain. When she was thrown out of it one day, an army officer ordered a carriage to be prepared.

Originally a baggage-wagon, when it was furnished with a comfortable seat, the size of a full length bed, and with a hood added, it resembled a baby's oversized perambulator. It had curtains to draw against bad weather and was drawn by two horses with a rider. Florence was so grateful and she rode in it for the rest of her stay in the Crimea.

On her travels she frequently witnessed blatant evidence of the futility of war. British, French and Russian soldiers who, only a matter of weeks before, had been trying to kill each other were now drinking together and organizing games.

Along with the troops, doctors and nurses were all preparing to leave the Crimea. Mother Bridgeman and her nurses sailed for England on 11th April. Shortly afterwards, Florence's favourite nurse, Mother Superior of the Bermondsey nuns, fell ill and she too had to be sent home.

When Florence had completed her inspection she returned to Scutari, determined to stay there until the last patient left the barracks hospital. The last patient left on 16th July.

Florence had been there for only twenty months but in that time she had personally been present at 2,000 deaths.

Of eight British Regiments, 75 per cent had perished or been maimed, and 250,000 lives had been lost by both sides, mostly through disease.

Despite being the best equipped force from the outset, only after the war ended was it discovered that the French army had experienced the highest sickness rate ever known in wartime.

Four months after the war ended, Florence and her aunt were offered berths aboard a naval battleship returning to England where all sorts of celebration awaited her.

Four Guards bands would greet her. Civic ceremonies had been arranged for whichever port she landed at, Folkestone or Dover. There would be triumphal arches, processions.

As her family was staying at Derbyshire, it was assumed she would go straight there so a man-drawn carriage was planned to take her from the railway station to Lea Hurst.

In view of the recent acclamation, Florence suspected as much so she settled instead for a civilian passenger vessel on which she and her aunt sailed under the names of Mrs and Miss Smith.

Disembarking at Marseilles they made their way to Paris for a short visit with Clarkey. Mai decided to stay on for a few days and Florence left for home alone.

What a reception awaited her in London. Just as she'd guessed, there were military bands, a hastily erected triumphal arch, a waving, cheering crowd and a welcoming committee.

When her train arrived at the platform, in all the excitement no one noticed the frail looking woman in dark clothes stepping out of an end carriage. And before people started to get suspicious of her non-appearance, she had slipped quietly away into the city and taken rooms for the night.

First thing next morning, Florence went to the Bermondsey convent to enquire about the Mother Superior. With the other nuns, they prayed thanks to God that the terrible carnage of the past two years was over. Florence stayed until the afternoon then set off to the station. By the time her whereabouts was discovered, she was already on a train making for Derbyshire.

From the station she walked along the lane and paused a while as her beloved Lea Hurst came into view, standing on its high rise. Moments later she was walking up the sweeping drive and into the house.

When Florence walked into the drawing-room her family, assuming she was being lauded in London, were shocked both at her unexpected arrival and at how pale and ill she looked. She was gaunt, her face so thin and pinched as to be barely recognizable. Her hair, though beginning to grow again, still looked severely cropped to them and it was easy to see how she'd managed to slip away unnoticed by the crowd.

When they asked why she'd evaded all the

publicity, Florence replied that she couldn't understand "all the fuzz-buzzy about my name".

11.

"I CAN NEVER FORGET"

There was a lot of fuss from her family though.
Florence was no longer the outcast they were
once ashamed of. All Britain was acclaiming her
a heroine and her mother and sister gloried in
her fame. Assuming she would soon be making
public appearances and giving interviews, they
encouraged her to rest in order to regain her
health and beauty in preparation for the celebrations.

They too would surely be involved in all the
publicity – what about a new wardrobe for them
all? Fanny and Parthe were asking. They
imagined themselves sitting on platforms,
receiving ovations, as much recipients of
the accolade as the Lady with the Lamp
herself.

Every day invitations came from Dukes, Earls
and Barons, offering their homes for Florence's
recuperation.

Artists wanted to paint her portrait. Gifts of
jewellery arrived. Gifts of silverware from
master cutlers. Masses of mail: letters of praise,

of thanks, begging letters and marriage proposals.

Though Parthe was helpful in answering them all on Flo's behalf, she still faced a dilemma. In her heart she wished Florence hadn't embarrassed the family by getting involved with nursing. Yet at the same time, although she disapproved of its source, she envied her sister's popularity and hoped it would reflect on to her. She was hoping too that now Flo was home, she would devote all her time to her.

But Florence had too much to think about and she could neither rest nor relax, much less confine her interests to her demanding sister.

There were so many things to do, her mind was buzzing.

Night after night she paced the floor in her bedroom trying to sort herself out. She wanted to nurse more than anything yet, for the past three years, what with Harley Street and Scutari, she'd been more an administrator. And now she should be free to return to nursing she was haunted by the memories of all the suffering she'd seen.

She wrote to the troops, "I am a bad mother to desert you and leave you in your Crimean graves."

"I can never forget" was a phrase that constantly ran through her mind. It appeared in her diary and at odd times when she was sitting, thinking about something else, her pen would wander across the page and always it left the same message: "I can never forget."

In the name of the men who had died, she knew she must go on fighting for improvements.

Thousands would have been saved had conditions been different. In wartime, wounds, maimings and deaths are inevitable but if only the terrible diseases could have been prevented.

She was determined that every aspect of soldiers' lives must be improved, especially their barracks and medical care. And there was no time to lose. Once war memories began to fade, the fickle public conscience would lose interest. Anything that could possibly be done must be set in motion straightaway. But how could she, a mere woman, take on the vast machine of the British Army?

She told Sidney Herbert, "There are people at the War Office who would burn me given the chance." The only possible way to achieve anything would be through a Royal Commission.

Then, in September, just as she had heard the Lord call to her at a time when everything seemed hopeless, she received an invitation from Sir James Clark, the family doctor who had once told her to get away from home when Parthenope had her breakdown.

He was asking her to come and recuperate

from her ordeal at his holiday home in Scotland. The Queen was in Scotland until the autumn. She wanted to meet Florence and his home, Birk Hall, was on the Balmoral estate.

Florence really wasn't well enough to face the 600-mile rail journey but she accepted, nevertheless. WEN went with her and they broke their journey at Edinburgh, supposedly for a rest, but Florence visited hospitals and an orphanage while she was there.

Her first audience with the Queen was very formal. Prince Albert was there and so was Lord Panmure, the new Secretary of State for War. He read out a letter thanking her "on behalf of himself and his colleagues and to express the unanimous feeling of the people of this country".

Afterwards the Queen gave her a private audience as she wanted to hear the full story of Scutari. Florence knew she must take advantage of the opportunity and had taken with her the enquiry's report on conditions at the barracks hospital. She showed it to the Queen and told her of her own plans for army reform.

The meeting lasted two hours. Both Queen Victoria and Prince Albert were very impressed by her. Later that evening when writing a letter to her Commander-in-Chief, the Duke of Cambridge – one of the committee that helped launch the Nightingale Fund – the Queen wrote,

"I wish we had her at the War Office."

Over the next week, Florence was invited to the castle every day. The Queen would turn up unexpectedly at Birk Hall and stay for tea. They went for long walks together through the woods while they discussed her plans.

Victoria herself had no direct power, but she had influence. At the end of Flo's stay in Scotland she promised to have a Royal Commission set up to enquire into the disgraceful conditions at Scutari and put forward Florence's recommendations for improvement.

Among these were: improvements to the army's sanitary conditions, training of army nurses, distribution of food and medical supplies. The transport system – particularly of sick and wounded – needed a complete overhaul. The most ambitious proposal was that a Military Hospital should be established in England.

The Royal Commission, with Sidney Herbert presiding as Chairman, was set up for the following year, 1857. Sidney Herbert suggested to Lord Panmure that, in the meantime, plans for the suggested hospital should be drawn up. That would show the public that the government was in favour of reforms.

Panmure agreed. A suitable location was found and when plans for the Netley Army Hospital were drafted, he sent them to Florence for approval – but she didn't approve. Everything about them was hopelessly out of date so she modified them and returned them to Panmure who promised to have them amended. But it was too late. Building had already commenced. Seventy thousand pounds worth of work had been done and nothing could be altered.

Feeling she'd been patronised in having her opinion sought for no reason, Florence complained to PAM, the Prime Minister, who instructed work to be stopped. The hospital was supposed to be for the welfare of soldiers, not as a monument to great architecture, he said.

Arguments raged between him and Lord Panmure but the Prime Minister lost. Netley Hospital was completed with just a few minor alterations that weren't affected by the work already done.

As time was drawing nearer for the Royal Commission to begin, Florence had a foreboding that it would never reach fruition. Members of Parliament, she knew, were quibbling among themselves, thinking up all manner of excuses for delay – and preferably for a cancellation.

To exercise some power of her own, she issued a threat to the government and the War Office. If the enquiry hadn't begun within three months' time she would go public and publish the full story of Scutari with all its bungling bureaucracy and incompetence.

Her threat proved successful and in May 1857,

the Royal Commission sat for the first time.

Florence moved to London and took a suite of rooms in the Burlington Hotel close to Whitehall, the hub of political activity.

Throughout the long, stifling summer, droves of experts, victims of the system, war victims and anyone else who could give vital information passed through her sitting-room, each giving invaluable advice and making valid suggestions.

Florence herself appeared at the Commission to give evidence.

From early morning until the early hours of the following day, she worked on the additional information she'd been given, compiling reports to pass on.

But she was never well. During the period in Turkey her constitution had been ruined both with the long hours she'd worked and with the nature of the work. The climate hadn't suited her either and she'd missed far more meals than she'd actually eaten. Reared in the bosom of a wealthy family and leading a life of luxury, waited on hand and foot by servants, nobody could have conceived that she would ever experience such hardships.

To add to the strain of her work and ill health, her mother and Parthe also moved into the hotel. It was early summer and the Season was just getting under way but they were prepared to sacrifice such pleasures in order "to take great care of her".

This they did by lying around on couches all day long. With skirts decorously arranged and delicately wafting fans, smelling salts to hand, each urged the other not to overtax her strength by arranging flowers in vases or by standing at the window too long looking down into the street.

Yet all the while, in the next room, Florence was punishing her frail body beyond its limits. She found their presence most irritating, particularly when they kept interrupting her train of thought over some trivial matter. She knew why her mother and sister were there and it wasn't to take care of her. But as she'd turned her back on all the "fuzz-buzzy" they were wasting their time.

When the hotel management let Parthe's room for the night by mistake, Flo was ordered to take the one offered in exchange and let her sister sleep in her room. She couldn't expect Parthe to be inconvenienced.

Her mother and sister had taken the carriage to London but Flo had to travel in hansom-cabs, omnibuses and trains.

Teams toured the country for information and Flo herself went from barracks to barracks, from hospital to hospital. On returning to the hotel late one night after a particularly strenuous day, her mother remarked, "What an amusing life you lead."

Florence was forever compiling statistics on general standards of cleanliness, diet, background, environment, ages, types of illness, deaths versus recoveries, treatment. Her aim was not so much to cure disease as to prevent it.

One of her favourite quotes was: "To understand God's thoughts we must study statistics, for these are the measure of his purpose."

To demonstrate the numbers of men who had died in hospital through poor hygiene and disease in comparison to deaths resulting from war wounds, she would take a round cottage loaf and cut it into wedges. Each section represented a percentage of those dying from cholera, typhus or gangrene; death from wounds; death following surgery. And always the largest wedge related to disease.

Thus Florence Nightingale invented the pie-chart.

All of this was dismissed as rubbish by sceptics. How could diseases be prevented when no one knew how they were caused in the first place?

Undaunted, Flo vowed to ensure conditions improved for British troops, not only in times of war but in peace-time too. On her tours up and down the country she'd discovered that living standards in England's barracks fell far short of what she considered minimum requirements. They were dark, airless, oppressive and dirty.

She wrote a 1,000-page document pointing out the necessity for extreme cleanliness in all things, and for good, nourishing food.

Army authorities and some politicians felt antagonized at a woman telling them what they ought to do. But though her voice was soft and her manner gentle, Florence could be quite formidable. And with the Queen showing interest and concern all the way, they were obliged to take note of every recommendation she made.

When the Commission's Report came out in August, the findings revealed what Florence had claimed all along. There was no lack of finances or supplies – medical or otherwise. All the problems facing the troops in the Crimean War were brought about by blatant bureaucracy and officiousness.

But rather than acknowledge the findings, the government – under her friend, Lord Palmerston – made all sorts of excuses, exonerating army officials and everybody else who'd been in authority.

Florence couldn't believe it. "Have they learned *nothing*?" she asked Sidney Herbert.

While waiting for the report she'd been getting low-spirited. Now her disappointment at the outcome added to her distress. What had been the point of all her research and reports if the results were being swept under the proverbial carpet?

Nothing had changed. Apart from the building of the Netley Military Hospital, which had turned out to be a fiasco, none of the improvements she'd recommended would be made. And if – or inevitably whenever – another war broke out, the same conditions she'd witnessed at Scutari would exist.

In a terrible state of depression, she began spending all her days in bed. This was partly from genuine illness but mainly to keep Fanny and Parthe at bay. Much as they claimed to be "taking care of her", they had no desire to visit a sick-room and she couldn't cope with them when she had so much on her mind.

Florence had no time for sleep or food and was living on tea. She became so weak that in August she collapsed. Everybody, including herself, thought she was dying.

After a couple of days she rallied a bit but wouldn't accept she'd been overworking. She needed some time alone, far away from her relatives, so she went to Malvern Spa in Worcestershire to take the mineral waters.

Her mother and sister left London for Derbyshire. WEN travelled down from Lea Hurst to see Flo and wrote home that she was dying.

But Fanny and Parthe said they couldn't bring themselves to go and see her.

Florence could scarcely breathe and talking was an effort. Night saw her lying awake, hour after hour, thinking, planning. By day she was writing though she could barely hold a pen and she was constantly summoning her "aides" to come up from London for consultations.

Much to her family's annoyance, once again aunt Mai stepped in and went to Malvern where she stayed until Flo had recovered enough to return to London. With Fanny and Parthe gone home, Florence felt a great sense of freedom and claimed she was ready to get on with her work.

She left the Burlington Hotel in favour of a suite of rooms at an hotel in Hampstead and gave her address to no one save a chosen few. In reality the few numbered hundreds.

Surrounded by a profusion of pet white Persian cats, she took permanently to her bed and saw no one except by appointment. Her five servants had strict instructions to keep unwelcome callers at bay. Visitors were by appointment only and were allowed thirty minutes with her and no longer.

Journalists were denied interviews and she absolutely refused to appear in public.

Again she was writing, writing, writing, every day, all day and well into the night.

She didn't neglect writing to close friends and

some relatives. Her father was included in this selected group and she wrote to him often but she would have nothing to do with either her mother or her sister.

Whenever they tried to contact her, if only by letter, she became so distressed her heart started pounding and sometimes she fainted, especially if they suggested going to visit her.

Most of her letter writing, however, was directed to anyone who could help in her struggle.

Florence knew now it was only through Parliament that the soldiers' welfare would be improved. From her studies of Parliamentary Reports in her early years she was familiar with all the offices and knew precisely who to approach for information. So she set about enrolling everybody in the Commons and the House of Lords who she thought might be sympathetic to her ideas. They had the power and she would harness it to her cause.

Sidney Herbert was her obvious first choice. She cajoled the rest into following and boldly stated what they must fight for, on her behalf. This group became known as her Cabinet. Like a queen holding court she received them round her bed.

Although Florence wouldn't see reporters she wrote to them, and to editors, airing her views and asking their opinions on them. She did it in such a way that in a matter of days articles on those very topics would appear in newspapers and other journals without the authors realizing they'd written them at her instigation.

Anyone she thought had influence she sent pamphlets, or more often, rough drafts of them, under the label of confidentiality. It never failed. People were so flattered at being singled out for their opinion, they invariably took up her cause.

Whenever a public appointment was coming vacant, Florence put forward to the appropriate quarters names of people sympathetic to her ideas. Gradually she was building up her own little empire. Behind every relevant question and proposition put to the Commons or the Lords, the thoughts of Miss Nightingale could be discerned.

The situation became such common knowledge that one of her Cabinet, Sir Henry Verney, was referred to by colleagues as the "Member of Parliament for Florence Nightingale".

Sir Henry was an extremely wealthy widower of fifty-six and father of four children. A generous man, he'd built a model village for tenants on his estate in Buckinghamshire and had founded schools. In a cholera outbreak at Aylesbury, he helped to nurse the victims. He was handsome and charming and Florence loved his company, but he took her by surprise one day by declaring that he loved her and wanted to take care of her. Would she marry him?

Florence nearly collapsed again from shock. She was thirty-seven by then. Richard Monckton Milnes was the only man she had ever loved and she'd rejected him to answer God's calling. Now that call was even more urgent.

When she refused Sir Henry's proposal he was terribly upset. Fanny heard about it and was so angry she invited him to go and stay at Embley Park to help get over the disappointment.

Florence continued trying to achieve as many of her proposed reforms as possible in the few years she believed were left to her. In spite of her aunt's pleas, she sometimes worked until she fainted from fatigue.

This self-imposed withdrawal from the world was an extremely difficult decision to make when she also needed the public's support.

As she'd predicted, with people grown accustomed to peace, memories of the Crimea were gradually fading and the vision of the Lady with the Lamp dimmed to obscurity as other topics took precedence.

At Westminster in London, a huge crack had been discovered in the new sixteen-and-a-half-ton clock tower bell – now Big Ben.

From farther afield came word that Dr Livingstone had completed his trek across Africa.

And on the sub-continent, there was talk of threatened mutiny in India. If mutiny erupted it meant the British army would be fighting again.

12

ST THOMAS'S – THE NIGHTINGALE TRAINING SCHOOL

Those were the days of the British Empire and, following the fall of the East India Company, the beginning of the British Raj. And India wasn't a happy country.

Lots of unpopular reforms were being introduced. Old customs and traditions were swept away. Plans were being made to give women more freedom. Land was being taken for roads and railways.

Some religious practices were banned, like *suttee*, the burning to death of a Hindu wife on her husband's funeral pyre.

After months of rumour and counter-rumour, the mutiny finally erupted at Meerut in northern India and quickly spread to Delhi.

The uprising was speedily quashed but inevitably with loss of life on both sides and public interest in the army awoke again.

Florence wanted to go out as she had to Scutari, but Sidney Herbert was adamant she shouldn't. For one thing, she wasn't fit enough, and secondly, he was ill himself. Florence had got him involved in all her work and it wouldn't be right to leave him with the burden.

He reasoned with her that by pushing forward plans for improvements she was helping the troops in India every bit as much as if she were there.

Florence acceded but she was irritated at his claim to ill health. They were mere "fancies". She was the one who was overworked and ill, dying even.

In her diary she wrote, "I stand at the altar of the murdered men and while I live I fight their cause."

Now her attention was focused on conducting extensive research into the conditions under which British troops lived in India.

She also turned her mind to civilian matters, investigating the living standards of India's poor. Florence had never been to India so all her information was acquired through personal correspondence, reports from returning army officers and their families, politicians, journalists and press photographers.

The enquiry uncovered such appalling conditions in the sub-continent that she proposed another Royal Commission be set up.

To put forward all the arguments in favour of it, she wrote a 2,000-page report divulging that India's hygiene, diet and sanitation were in a diabolical state.

Always at Florence's side, her adoring aunt Mai helped a lot, mostly dealing with correspondence. But at times, although Sidney Herbert was now Minister *for* War, Florence treated him as though he were her personal secretary.

Helping compile statistics, checking reports, taking dictation, he was being pushed beyond endurance. But Florence, thoughtless – perhaps ruthless – seemed blind to everything except the completion of what they'd begun. Whenever Sidney appeared before her, bowed and weary, she never failed to remind him that *she* was the invalid.

In the previous year when Sir Henry Verney went to Embley Park to get over Florence rejecting his marriage proposal, he turned for consolation to Parthenope. And in April 1858, they announced their intention to marry.

Fanny was overjoyed. Parthe was turned forty so Fanny had resigned herself to both her daughters ending their lives as spinsters like her own sister, Julia, and her niece Hilary.

The forthcoming nuptials incurred a grand spending spree so she, Parthe and Hilary Bonham-Carter went to London, shopping for the trousseau. But they didn't venture to go near Florence and stayed at a different hotel.

In the June, Parthe became Lady Verney and moved from her parents' home to her new residence, palatial Claydon House in Buckinghamshire, about seventy-five miles away.

After her marriage, with no rivalry now between them, there was a big change in Parthe's relationship with her sister and they became much closer. Still Flo refused to have anything to do with her mother.

Sidney Herbert was worse and in the August he went to Ireland for a long holiday. In his absence Flo continued preparing work in readiness for when he came home, but when they got back to London Liz told her he had a serious kidney complaint and was also suffering dreadfully from neuralgic pains in his head. She hinted that he should really ease up on work.

Florence was quite unsympathetic and told Liz it was *she* who was dying "yet *he* complains of a headache".

By the November, Florence was so sure she was on the point of death she sent for Sidney and Parthe. He was to witness her last Will and Testament and Parthe was to arrange her funeral.

But death didn't come. In 1859 she became deeply engrossed in the Indian Sanitary Commission.

After India she turned her attention to civilian and maternity hospitals in Britain whose standards of hygiene were almost lethal.

Numerous pamphlets were written and that year she produced her book *Notes on Hospitals*.

This gave concise directions for building construction, hospital management, administration and improved sanitation.

When wards had four rows of beds crammed together, Florence recommended they should have only two rows placed against opposite walls with plenty of space between. On either side of the ward should be long casement windows, preferably one behind each bed. To preserve human dignity, every ward should have portable screens for placing round each bed.

These and other similar innovations – which today we take for granted – were revolutionary for the time but the book sold in thousands all over the world.

They could do nothing about their existing buildings but every London hospital, and many outside the capital, adopted her methods and standards of hygiene and agreed to the need to keep statistics. Soon after, Holland and Portugal approached Florence for advice about their own hospitals.

Later that year a follow-up book *Notes on Nursing* was published. It was an expensive publication at 5s (25p), yet it sold even more copies worldwide – 15,000 in the first month – and was translated into several languages.

The book didn't teach nursing techniques but concentrated on the *art* of nursing. It was full of sensible advice such as giving patients hot sweet drinks for shock, when it was a common belief that a piece of dry bread was best.

She enthused over the benefits of sunlight and fresh air – at that time, fresh air was associated with being cold and sunlight was bad for the sick. They were usually kept in darkened rooms.

Regarding diet, patients should be given lots of fruit and vegetables rather than just bland pap.

Great attention was paid to both a nurse's personal cleanliness and that of her patients and everything that came into contact with them: wards, bedding, kitchens, eating utensils, operating theatres, medical instruments and dressings.

Care of patients should be put above all other considerations, and not merely their physical well being. Washing, feeding and tending bodies weren't all that nursing involved. Their emotions were equally important.

How wretched patients felt when they knew doctors were talking over their case just out of earshot, leaving them anxious and wondering. She advocated telling them what was wrong, what to expect and what treatment.

While Florence was utterly opposed to women leading idle lives and to their being treated as chattels, in her book she made it clear they shouldn't aspire to the traditional male roles. The idea of female doctors, lawyers or Members of Parliament was as abhorrent to her as to anyone at that time.

By their very nature women should serve and be supportive of men, but they should be given their due respect.

Ludicrous though it seems today, Florence also felt the need to stipulate that nurses should be "good women" and not drunks with immoral or criminal tendencies.

The verdict on the *Notes on Nursing* was given by someone as "They have taught ladies how to be nurses and nurses how to be ladies".

In that same year, St Thomas's Hospital in London became involved in controversy when the South Eastern Railway Company announced its intentions to build a new railway line. Running from London Bridge to Charing Cross it was on a direct route for the hospital. A decision had to be made whether to demolish the old building and sell the company the whole site, or to stay and sell only part of it.

The matron of St Thomas's was a personal friend of Florence's and suggested that the chief medical officer seek her opinion. He did and was advised that the hospital be moved to a new building on a different site.

Florence was now forty. Ever since returning from Turkey she'd had it in the back of her mind to establish a Training School for Nurses. Until now there had been nowhere suitable but a new

St Thomas's could give her the opportunity she'd been waiting for.

The Nightingale Fund presented to her by the British public had risen to £50,000 – only four doctors had subscribed to it, yet £9,000 was donated from soldiers forgoing one day's pay. With a substantial sum like that and a brand new hospital in which to house it, Florence saw the fulfilment of her dreams beckoning.

As was expected, she was consulted about the hospital design and from then on supervised every aspect of its founding.

Marianne Nicholson had never forgiven Florence for hurting her brother, Henry. There was still a distance between them but Marianne's husband, Captain Douglas Galton, was a brilliant construction engineer and Florence wasn't about to let family discord stand in her way.

Captain Galton was brought into the organization and he and Florence were constantly conferring with builders, architects, designers, interior designers and ironmongers.

The wards were built precisely to her design. She was even consulted about sinks, cooking-pots and pans, glassware, crockery, cutlery and linen.

The hospital was opened in June 1860 and was the first ever to have a training scheme for nurses. The Nightingale Training School was housed on the whole of an upper floor and nurses were given their own rooms. This was the forerunner of what were later to become Nurses Homes.

Through the Fund, the School was financed independently from the rest of the hospital and the matron from the old St Thomas's Hospital, Mrs Wardroper, was made Superintendent. She was a woman from Florence's own social class who had only taken up nursing as a widow of forty-two.

Until then, nurses had been controlled and given work schedules by doctors but were never medically trained. There was a common fallacy that it was unnecessary as women were born with a natural ability to nurse, emanating from their maternal instinct. What bit of knowledge they picked up was from watching physicians on wards and surgeons at the operating-table – and of course, there were no female doctors then.

Florence had always maintained nurse training should be undertaken by women and she had immense faith in Mrs Wardroper. Nevertheless, all lessons and lectures were personally planned by Florence and she chose the students.

The trainees were given attractive brown uniform dresses with white aprons and caps. They had free food, bed and laundry and were given

£10 a year for personal expenses. Training was for one year, their tuition including the duties of a matron and a Superintendent.

Mostly the school produced matrons, for Florence had always intended its purpose being to teach nurse tutors who would then go out into the world, open their own establishments and train others.

She needed to know each individual trainee so they were amongst the very few people she entertained at her home when they came for afternoon tea.

They were instructed to keep a daily journal of all their activities and to produce it for her perusal at the end of each month.

Usually women drawn into nursing were ignorant and illiterate, mere carers in a very basic way. But in 1856 one doctor had said it was essential that they should be literate. Florence didn't believe a high standard of education was necessary, but she did agree nurses should at least be able to read and write.

All this involvement had been conducted from her bed and had sapped Florence of the little energy she had. Now she was so weak as to be unable to stand. Sometimes she would be carried from her bedroom to the sitting-room and placed on a day bed.

In 1861, when the Hospital and the Training School were well established, everybody, particularly aunt Mai, hoped she would take some rest.

But William Howard Russell, *The Times* war correspondent, was in America reporting on the Civil War and British readers were taking a keen interest in events. Recalling his Crimean reports, the authorities in America approached Florence for advice on sanitary organization and administration in the Northern States hospitals. So again she was writing from morning until the early hours of the following day.

That year, Queen Victoria offered her a "grace and favour" apartment in Kensington Palace but Florence graciously declined. She needed to be in the city where she still received her "Cabinet" almost daily.

If Florence believed it was a woman's place to serve men, she didn't apply that theory to Sidney Herbert. She constantly urged him on, and he gave her his full support while his wife and everyone around him could see he wasn't fit to continue.

Eventually, he had to tell her he was mortally ill but if he retired he could live a little longer. Still, she insisted he carry on.

But finally he was forced to resign from office and was created a Baron, taking the title of Lord Herbert of Lea. Even then Florence was very reproachful, implying that he'd let her down.

At his country seat, Wilton House in

Wiltshire, Sidney Herbert died on 2nd August 1861. His last thoughts were of the Lady with the Lamp and his dying words were, "Poor Florence! Poor Florence! Our joint work unfinished. I have tried to do my best."

Florence was utterly devastated when she heard the news and refused to see anyone. She saw all the reforms she'd fought so hard to implement slipping from her grasp.

In her diary she wrote, "My work, the object of my life, the means to it, all in one, depart."

For someone so steeped in compassion, it appears uncharacteristic for her to react to his death by bemoaning the fact she had lost "the means to it . . ." without giving a thought to him personally.

Sidney Herbert, she claimed, had taken her life with him – as work was her life. Her greatest supporter, he who had wielded so much power in the government was no more and she felt he'd no right to die, leaving her at a crucial time.

Now she believed her life was at an end – or at least, the effective part of it – and she felt bereft with only her profusion of cats and aunt Mai for company.

Florence became quite paranoid. Letters to close associates complained that she had ailed for twenty-five years and no one cared. Now she was so weak she was barely able to write.

All the same, reclining in her bed, she began

working as hard as ever. Now her attention was
turned to the poverty-stricken and the unedu-
cated.

At the insistence of her family, after nearly
three years' absence, aunt Mai decided to return
home to Derbyshire. Florence was furious at her
desertion and vowed never to speak to her
again, even though Mai had arranged for Hilary
Bonham-Carter to come and replace her as companion and secretary.

Hilary had made a niche for herself in the art
world as a talented painter and sculptor. And
although Flo hated any "fuzz-buzzy", within
weeks of her cousin moving in, she conde-
scended to let her sculpt a bust of her.

Florence and Hilary had always been fond of
each other and neither had ever married so their
new domestic arrangements appeared to be
ideal. However, in this instance, Florence
showed more sympathy than she had towards
her mentor, Sidney Herbert. She didn't feel it
right that Hilary should sacrifice her career to
either herself or her obligations so she sent her
home.

Meanwhile, events in the north of England
were about to draw the name of Florence Nightingale into yet another organization.

William Rathbone, a wealthy Liverpool merchant, had recently lost his wife despite the
good care of a local woman, Mary Robinson.

For months afterwards, William couldn't stop thinking of her excellent care so, to show his gratitude, he offered to pay Mary a good weekly wage and supply her with all the necessary equipment if she would take up nursing the sick in poorer parts of the city.

But the demand was too great. Conditions in the slums weren't conducive to good health and Mary was nursing as many sick people as there were fit ones walking about.

William Rathbone then asked the Board at Liverpool Royal Infirmary if they would be interested in starting a training school similar to the one he'd heard of in London – but with the aim of putting nurses into people's homes rather than into hospitals.

When Florence was consulted about the proposed scheme she heartily endorsed it and offered all the necessary advice.

William Rathbone financed the whole project, buildings, equipment and uniforms. And a newly-trained Nightingale Nurse, Miss Merryweather, was hired as matron/tutor.

The first nurses began work in private homes in late 1861 and became the District Nursing Service we have today. By 1887 nearly every city in Great Britain had its District Nurses.

13.

THE LAMP EXTINGUISHED

In Switzerland in 1863, after a young banker, Henri Durant, had finished reading about the Lady with the Lamp he couldn't get out of his mind all she'd achieved for the men at Scutari. But, he thought, there must have been hundreds if not thousands more whom she couldn't help: prisoners of war, even enemy soldiers. No one knew what conditions they'd contended with.

It worried him so much he was prompted to write a book suggesting a universal organization be set up to give access to all fighting men, irrespective of creed, race or politics. It could provide food where there was a shortage, arrange communication between prisoners and their families, and provide all manner of aid and comfort.

The book sold all over the world and in 1864 fourteen nations signed the Geneva Convention relating to treatment of prisoners. The organisation became the Red Cross. And although Florence hadn't been actively involved in establishing it, because she had been its source of inspiration, she was asked to take control of the British branch.

Two years later, after being instrumental in the founding of District Nursing, William Rathbone heard of the appalling conditions existing in a Liverpool city workhouse. Again he applied for assistance – this time directly to St Thomas's Hospital.

Twelve nurses, under the guidance of matron Agnes Jones, travelled north and found the workhouse in a similar state to what Florence found at the Barracks Hospital in Scutari.

Sick paupers – 15,000 of them – were caring for each other as best they could. Supervisors wore leather gloves to avoid touching anything, inmates included, and police patrolled the wards at night.

Agnes Jones and her nurses revolutionized the place and similar schemes for workhouses were introduced in London. This move was instrumental in the Poor Law Act being reformed.

True to character, Florence then added workhouses and workhouse hospitals to her list of concerns.

That same year, her father bought her a pleasant house with a large garden in South Street, Mayfair, London – and Hilary Bonham-Carter died of cancer.

Florence was as much angry as grieved at Hilary's death. She had been a slave to her family, sacrificing her art and her entire life to their care. "There but for the grace of God go I," she thought.

In August the following year, Parthe told Florence their mother was very ill. She'd had a coach accident in which she'd been heavily thrown, sustaining bruising and shock.

For some time Florence had known her mother was going blind but they'd been estranged for so long, ever since Fanny left the Burlington when Flo went to Malvern. She hadn't been near Embley Park, not even for Parthe's wedding, nor had she visited her beloved Lea Hurst.

Now Fanny was too ill to travel nearly 200 miles from Embley to Derbyshire for the autumn but WEN had to go there on business.

As Parthe's husband, Sir Henry, was a Member of Parliament and she now a popular society hostess, they lived mostly at their London home and she couldn't leave for Embley. So WEN implored Flo to go and stay with her mother.

For the fifty-mile journey, she travelled in an invalid carriage. Only some of her servants went with her but she took all of the documents she was working on.

In the nine years since they'd met, Fanny, at

seventy-eight, had changed considerably. When Florence saw the struggle she had to focus her failing sight on her daughter, a great surge of regret swept through her and they greeted each other warmly.

An entire floor of the house had been prepared for her sole use. With her servants and her stack of papers she took up residence there and never moved out of the rooms except to be carried to see her mother in hers.

Fanny spent her days in bed and took a carriage drive in the evenings. Her change of character was remarkable. But servants who hadn't seen Florence for almost a decade were remarking on the change in her character too.

It was as though mother and daughter had undergone a role reversal for now, at forty-six, it was Florence who was difficult and demanding. No one dared refuse her anything or disagree with what she said. Apart from her mother, the only ones she could relate to were children and grandchildren of the many cousins when they visited the great house.

In October, WEN returned home and Flo went back to London.

Among her next projects was a training programme suggested by Parthe's husband for some health missionaries at Buckinghamshire – the Health Visitors we know today.

That was followed by a three-year study of

health care for young mothers and their babies from the poorer classes.

During the Franco-German war in 1870 Florence was approached by both sides for advice on medical matters. After the war, France awarded her with the bronze cross of the Societe de Secours aux Blesses. From Germany she received the Cross of Merit.

By then, Nightingale-trained nurses had founded schools as far away as America and Australia. Training schools had sprung up all over Britain and still more Nightingale nurses were needed. In 1872 St Thomas's was undergoing a massive building project to expand its school and, once more, Florence was called in.

She considered moving house to be nearby while the extensions were being made, but then Parthe told her their father and mother were both ill. Fanny was aged eighty-three, WEN, seventy-seven. Parthe couldn't go to them as she was suffering from arthritis and could barely walk.

Florence went to Embley and was no sooner there than the elderly housekeeper died. The young servants knew little of what was expected of them so she took over the household organization with the same relish she had shown at Scutari.

Fanny was becoming childish, weeping and fretting a lot, so Florence decided she must stay there. Slowly she felt herself being drawn back into the net. Her mother was demanding. Parthe, selfish as ever, was living like a princess in London. As with Sidney Herbert, Florence couldn't accept that her sister was ill.

After eight months she had to return home to attend to the St Thomas's extension programme. Worried about her parents, she decided to take her mother with her and arranged for aunt Julia, Fanny's younger spinster sister, to move into Embley and take care of WEN.

Absolutely worn out, Florence arrived home to find waiting for her communications requesting information and advice from the War Office, India, hospitals, orphanages, workhouses, training schools. For the first time in her life, it was too much.

"This year I go out of office!" she declared and announced her intention to retire.

It was strange that, in all her life, the only thing she had ever really longed to do was nurse. Yet of all the work over the years, only at odd times in her year at Harley Street and during her first few weeks at Scutari had she actually been a nurse.

In an effort to redress the irony of her non-nursing career, she planned to give up her May-fair home and live in a hospital for the rest of her days. With this in mind, when her mother was a little better, she took her back to Embley but Fanny was so ill when they arrived, again she had to stay.

Constantly depressed now she retreated to her rooms and tried to overcome it by writing pamphlets on India, essays on religion and philosophy, and some Bible stories for children.

Just after Christmas, as the arthritis pain had eased slightly and Parthe was feeling a little better, she and her husband turned up at Embley. They intended staying for quite a while so it gave Florence the opportunity to go home – just in time to hear the first stirrings of what, in a few years' time, would be labelled the Battle of the Nurses.

There were two factions. One believed there should be a set training course for nurses, followed by practical and written examinations culminating in the participants becoming Registered Nurses. But Florence was opposed to registration believing it would turn nursing into a profession and thus rob it of a sense of vocation or calling.

She advised her students that certificates and diplomas weren't the objective of their training. Any nurse resting on those laurels was no nurse at all. Primary concerns should be the welfare of patients and to constantly improve on practical knowledge.

A week after she'd arrived home, on 10th January, 1874, she got word that her father had died in a tragic accident. When he got dressed that morning he'd forgotten to put his watch in his pocket so, while waiting for breakfast to be served, he went to get it. Coming downstairs, his sight at seventy-four not as sharp as it used to be, he'd tripped and tumbled to the bottom, dying instantly.

All her life Florence had shared a more loving relationship with him than with either her mother or her sister. The strongest bond was severed and she was crushed.

Living as a near recluse for so long was taking its toll of her. So many were dead, dying or grown feeble in mind and body. Yet she still believed it was she who was dying. Depression, the curse of her life, completely enveloped her. She felt the world had turned against her rather than admitting it was she who'd rejected it. In middle age she was beginning to crave company but it seemed there would soon be no one except her precious cats left for companionship.

As ever, she was quickly dragged out of her mental morass by all sorts of legal wrangling.

As a young man, WEN had been obliged to change his name from Shore to Nightingale in order to inherit his uncle's property. Now, through complicated relationships and clauses in his uncle's Will, both properties, Lea Hurst and Embley, passed to his sister, aunt Mai.

This brought a reconciliation between herself

and Florence after almost twenty years. But other than the satisfaction of knowing her son, Shore, would one day inherit it, the legacy was of little interest to Mai.

Florence, however, asked her to move into Embley thus enabling Fanny, aged ninety-two, to stay in her own home for the rest of her days. But Mai, herself nearing eighty, had no intention of moving house and Fanny was too infirm to stay on at Embley.

The solution was to move Fanny into South Street with Florence who was being increasingly drawn into Indian concerns. Once more she was "soaked in work".

For years, she'd been trying to get her father to improve the sewage and wells at Lea Hurst but he always maintained they were quite adequate. When in 1878 a typhus epidemic broke out in the village, the tenants blamed Florence because none of the work she'd suggested had been done. But as the estate didn't belong to her, it wasn't her responsibility.

Clarkey was staying in London at the time so, leaving Fanny in her charge, Florence went off to Derbyshire to try to put things right. The business took longer than she'd anticipated and she was there for weeks.

Clarkey wrote asking her to come home. Her mother had gone completely senile. She didn't know anybody or know where she was and kept calling for "Flo". Florence wrote that she couldn't get away for the next few days.

Then Parthe wrote, saying it was urgent and she must return to London.

Angrily, Florence replied, "Do you really think I'm here because I want to be? Do you think I've ever, in my life, been able to do anything I've really wanted to do? Every time it appeared that I would, my life was called on to do something entirely different."

Two days later another letter came from Clarkey. After listening to her favourite hymns all evening, Fanny had died peacefully in her sleep – while Florence was attending to the drains in Derbyshire.

She wasn't given much time to mourn for her mother. There was always India. She was now recognized as an expert on the country, the land, its people, health matters, law, education, its flora and fauna even, and every week brought more and more enquiries.

Always, always working, India apart, among what might be called incidental matters, she was asked to choose army nurses for Egypt.

Parthe was suffering terribly and so badly crippled that, like her sister, she had to be carried from place to place.

Sir Henry, retired from Parliament, and Parthe, now seventy-two and long since retired from being a society hostess, lived mainly at their grand home in Buckinghamshire. On the odd occasion when the Verneys were in London, Parthe had taken to visiting Florence at South Street every Sunday for tea.

On one visit, after being carried into the drawing-room and laid on a sofa, she said she wanted to stay until evening. When it was time to leave she asked to be taken home to Claydon House rather than to their London residence. Florence and Sir Henry pleaded with her against the fifty-mile drive. It was too much for her, particularly at that time of day, but Parthe was insistent.

A week later she was dead.

After her death, Florence and Sir Henry became inseparable companions and were positively devoted to each other. She spent so much time there that rooms were always held in readiness for her.

Sir Henry was eighty-nine but still an active and handsome man. Flo at seventy no longer believed she was at death's door.

Grown fat, hair grey, her eyes looked small in the sagging flesh, yet traces of her former beauty were still in evidence. Her health improved so much that every day she and Sir Henry strolled arm in arm through the grounds. On fine days they sat in the gardens until dusk. They were so dependent on each other that Florence came closer to him than to anyone in her life.

She still found it easy to relate to children and to the youngest of her Nightingale Nurse trainees. It was almost as though she adopted them as the children she'd never had and gave them pet names, often the names of her departed cats. As if it were her own home, she frequently invited them to Claydon House for weekends.

Her sight was beginning to go and her writing becoming more than just a physical effort. She strained to see it.

Officials from the various organizations she was involved with noticed the change in her handwriting and in the content of her work. It was evident her skills were diminishing. The time had come to stop burdening her with their problems. It seemed Florence was finding peace and rest at last.

Sir Henry Verney died in February 1894 aged 93. Flo never went back to Claydon House though his family were loving towards her and always asking "aunt Florence" to visit them.

In 1897 the British Empire was celebrating Queen Victoria's Jubilee. At seventy-eight, one year younger than Florence, she had been sixty years on the throne.

A great exhibition "The Victorian Era" was to depict all the achievements and great events of the age. One section was reserved to represent nursing with Miss Nightingale as the focal point of interest.

Florence was asked to loan a portrait of herself and photographs and relics of the Crimean war along with her sculpted bust.

She replied with vigour that the relics of the Crimean War were to be found in deaths, disease, ignorance and poor hygiene. The whole idea of "canonising" her was absurd, "and I've never had a portrait painted in my life".

One relic of the Crimean War did appear at the Exhibition. It was the carriage she'd ridden in during her final inspection at Balaklava. After the war, Alexis Soyer, her faithful chef, had had it shipped home and someone had found it in bits in an out-house at Embley. Re-assembled and cleaned up, it took pride of place in the Exhibition's section on nursing.

Since she had lived such a reclusive life over the past years, although the general public hadn't forgotten her, most believed she was dead. Generations born, grown and aged since the Crimean War had only dim recollections of hearing about the Lady with the Lamp. The Exhibition renewed flagging interest and, overnight, once again Florence Nightingale became a living legend.

Nearing eighty years of age, her sight now quite dim, she was appreciating the joy of living more than at any time in her life.

As more years went by, her mind began playing tricks on her. She'd completely retired from the world and knew little of what was going on around her. Those attending to her, she fancied, were people from her past calling to see her.

Sometimes, perhaps reliving the frustrations of Scutari, she shouted and issued orders.

From time to time, all manner of honours were heaped on her. Among others, they came from the Crimean Veterans and Red Cross Societies.

In 1907, aged eighty-seven, Florence was granted the Order of Merit, the first woman ever to be so honoured. By then her mind was wandering and confused. Much of her time was spent dozing in her chair or in bed.

When the honour was bestowed upon her at her London home, Sir Douglas Dawson made a small speech commending her for her good works. Florence was in bed, propped up in a cloud of pillows. She scarcely knew what was happening until he stooped and placed the medal in her hand. Then she was aware that something had been presented to her and was heard to murmur, "Too kind. Too kind."

In 1908 she was granted the Freedom of the City of London. The Roll was brought to her for signature but Florence didn't understand. Her hand was guided and she managed to write a simple FN.

At noon on 13th August, 1910, Florence Nightingale received her final call from God and fell into her last sleep. A grand funeral procession followed by burial in Westminster Abbey was offered – but Florence had requested that her body be donated to scientific research. No one would agree to that.

She was interred at the village churchyard in East Wellow, a village close to Embley Park, her old family home on the edge of the New Forest in Hampshire.

It was a very private occasion. Her bearers were six army sergeants.

There is no ostentatious monument. Florence could never understand all the "fuzz-buzzy" about her name. A simple gravestone reads:

FN Born 1820. Died 1910

EPILOGUE

Between 1860–1903, 2,000 nurses graduated from the Nightingale Training School.

By 1880 nursing had become a respectable vocation, even for ladies.

There is hardly a town or city in Great Britain where at least one hospital wasn't founded by a Nightingale Nurse. Many hospitals proudly display framed letters from Florence herself expressing her good wishes to the "matron".

After Florence's death her diaries, notes, letters, plans, statistics and papers on every aspect of her life were found scattered throughout the house. Drawers, cupboards, boxes, bags, coalscuttles, ornaments – every conceivable receptacle was filled. And it's from this vast amount of information that so many biographies have been compiled on the Lady with the Lamp.